GN01005804

MENOPAUSE
A Well Woman Book

MENOPAUSE
A WELL WOMAN BOOK

by

The Montreal Health Press

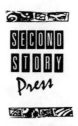

SECOND STORY Press

CANADIAN CATALOGUING IN PUBLICATION DATA

Gerson, Miryam,
   Menopause : a well woman book

Rev. ed. of: A book about menopause.
ISBN 0-929005-10-4

1. Menopause – Popular works. 2. Middle aged
women – Health and hygiene. I. Title. II.Title:
A book about menopause.

RG186.G47 1990   612.6'65   C90-093911-7

Copyright © 1990 by Montreal Health Press Inc.

Printed and bound in Canada

Published by
SECOND STORY PRESS
585½ Bloor Street West
Toronto, Canada
M6G 1K5

CONTENTS

THE MONTREAL HEALTH PRESS

Principal Writer	Miryam Gerson
Writers and Contributors	Rosemary Byrne-Hunter Marilyn Bicher Donna Cherniak Judith Crawley Shirley Pettifer
Illustrators	Michel Hébert pages 28, 49, 170, 171 Anne Massicotte pages 30, 31, 65, 74, 76, 102/3, 110, 176/7
Cover Photograph	Judith Crawley
Supporting Roles	Diane Comley Janet Torge Eileen Young

PHOTOGRAPHY CREDITS
(in order of first appearance)

PAMELA HARRIS *pages 10, 40, 165*
JUDITH CRAWLEY *pages 42, 71, 107, 140, 155, 184, 191*
ALAIN CHAGNON *pages 16, 89*
VINCENZO PIETROPAOLO *pages 18, 19, 37*
ANDRÉ BOURBONNAIS *pages 22, 24, 59, 90, 93*
BRENDA SPIELMANN *pages 34, 82*
ANITA PETITCLERC *pages 44, 146*
HELEN WHITEHEAD *page 47*
JOHN KAYSER *page 55*
ALAIN DÉCARIE *pages 63, 75*
LOUISE DE GROSBOIS *pages 85, 92*
CHERYL MEDICOFF *page 100*
DENISE SIROIS *page 115*
NESSA BEDWARD *page 123*
DEREK OSS *pages 126, 148, 159*
ANNICK BRENIEL *page 133*
ANNERIE VAN GEMERDEN *page 153*
CHARLES GAUTHIER *page 183*
DENISE FAILLE *pages 14, 182*
STAN ADAMS *page 169*

ACKNOWLEDGMENTS

Many people helped and supported us in the process of writing this book and in our first effort at paperback publication. The Health Promotion Directorate of Health and Welfare Canada recognized the unmet need of midlife women for information about menopause, and provided us with important financial support to write the book. Susan Dann, our project manager from Health and Welfare challenged us and critiqued our work, but always supported and encouraged us.

We offer special thanks to the women who generously agreed to be interviewed at the start of the project, and who sensitized us to the important issues of menopause.

Thanks as well, to all those who helped in production of *Menopause: A Well Woman Book,* including technical advisors, proofreaders and office staff.

Finally, we wish to thank the women at Second Story Press who have led us through the publication process with enthusiasm and patience. They have shown great respect for both our history as a group and our vision of women's health.

PREFACE

For those of us who have been involved in the women's health movement in Canada, the work of the Montreal Health Press has been like a wise older sister — there when you need her and always with the information you've been looking for. But like the wise older sister, we sometimes take her for granted. For over 20 years, during a period when we have seen the development of health groups and collectives, improved access to women's health services and a growing awareness of women's health issues at various government levels, the women at the Press have worked diligently at raising our awareness about our bodies and our health. They have done this on the basis of a deep respect for a woman's ability to make her own choices, once she is given the information she needs. By using an accessible format, they have succeeded in reaching a broad range of women. With the use of eloquent photographs, diagrams and clear language, they have helped to demystify the world of medicine and bring women's health issues to the forefront of the women's movement.

Just as they were there for us when we needed information about birth control, sexually transmitted diseases and sexual assault, they are here for us again with information about menopause. And for those of us who "grew up" with their material — many of us now reaching our menopausal years — this is a most welcome addition.

Their timing, as usual, is fortuitous. As a large group of women born in the post-war years approach this chapter in their life, they are being showered with information about menopause. Unfortunately, much of it has an underlying message: menopause is a time of crisis and hormone replacement therapy is the best solution. Pharmaceutical companies are putting large sums of money into advertisements aimed at convincing menopausal women to ask their doctors how they can help them, while simultaneously advertising to the doctors about the benefits of hormone replacement therapy. Headlines of newspaper columns by prominent physicians tell us that "menopause problems can be potentially serious," immediately establishing a climate of fear and worry in women readers. Menopause is treated as an illness or a disease, as something to be "gotten rid of," and women are left feeling that they are somehow irresponsible if they don't run to their doctor at the first signs of changes.

In sharp contrast, *Menopause: A Well Woman Book* is a clear and simple road map for women in their middle years who, while experiencing a very normal change, may find themselves in unknown territory. It acknowledges that the experience of menopause, like menstruation, childbirth and other stages of the life cycle, is highly individual. For some women it will be rough, for others, a breeze; there will be every potential variation in between those two extremes. Some will do well with hormones; for others, it simply is not neccessary. The Montreal Health Press presents a wealth of information in an non-prescriptive and non-judgemental style — a breath of fresh air in this artificially created climate of fear and anxiety. It has always been a major tenet of the women's health movement that information is empowering and that women know their bodies best. If given the full range of information, women will make the choices that are best for them.

This book reminds us that the best source of information about women's bodies is other women. We listen to our older sister who has already been there, and we learn to trust ourselves.

— Anne Rochon Ford
Toronto, 1990

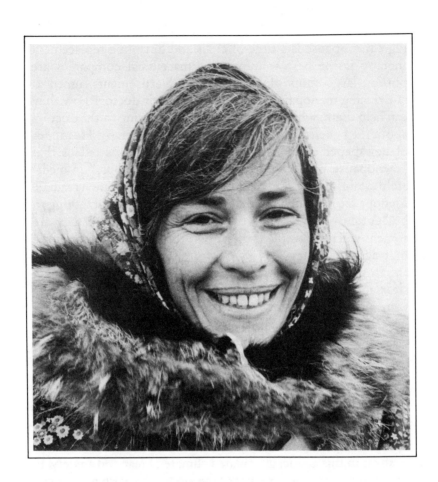

INTRODUCTION

Menopause: A Well Woman Book provides basic information about the experience of menopause. It explains, simply and clearly, what menopause is and why it happens. It describes the changes that can take place in a woman's body and suggests ways of dealing with them.

This book also looks at the stage of life in which menopause occurs. It discusses a variety of social and political issues that affect the health and wellbeing of mid-life women.

Menopause is a normal and natural process, yet many women are frightened by its approach. The subject is still sufficiently taboo that younger women are deprived of the opportunity to learn from older women. Negative stereotypes of menopause and of mid-life women still abound.

Menopause is an example of a normal life transition being turned into a disease. Through the medicalization of menopause we have lost our perspective on the reality of the experience and have lost confidence in what we can do on our own to keep ourselves healthy both physically and emotionally. Doctors rather than women are considered the experts on menopause, and the pharmaceutical companies reap the benefits. Ironically, women with money or access to medical services are more likely to be overtreated, while other women go without basic health care.

We are aware that many women do have a bad time at menopause, and often their distress can be relieved by medical treatment. However we are concerned about the generalization of treatment to all women. Not enough is known about the long-term effects, particularly regarding hormone therapy, to justify making guinea pigs out of a generation of women.

In *Menopause: A Well Woman Book* we have tried to strengthen women's confidence in our own abilities to deal with menopause. We have tried to avoid telling you what is best for you and what decisions you should make. We present different sides of the issues like hormone replacement therapy and hysterectomy, and point out areas in which the answers still are not known. We describe the social, political and economic factors that influence the different points of view.

This book is addressed to all women and can be used in different ways. It can prepare younger women for what to expect, and can give women in the middle of menopause a basis for comparison. It can be read straight through to give an overview of the experience or used as a reference book to look up specific questions. This book will be useful to health workers and educators, and to women involved with menopause self-help groups. It can also help men who would like to better understand the experience of menopause or provide support to the mid-life women in their lives.

The Montreal Health Press has been publishing materials on health and sexuality for 20 years. It has become our tradition to offer our readers not only accurate information, but also support and encouragement in their quest to become active and informed decision-makers around their own lives and health.

EXPLODING THE MYTHS OF MENOPAUSE

MYTH	CHAPTER
• Menopause is a disease.	*Part1:* The Politics of Menopause
• Women go crazy at menopause.	*Part 2:* Beyond the Big Four
• After menopause, a woman has no sex hormones.	*Part 4:* Sexuality at Mid-life and Beyond
• Hormone therapy keeps you young.	*Part 2:* General Body Changes
• Once a woman's periods are irregular, she cannot get pregnant anymore.	*Part 4:* Sexuality at Mid-life and beyond.
• More women get depressed around menopause than at any other time.	*Part 2:* Beyond the Big Four
• When a woman has a hysterectomy, her periods stop and she is finished with menopause.	*Part 3:* Hysterectomy and Surgical Menopause
• A woman taking hormones does not need birth control because the hormones are the same as in the birth control pill.	*Part 4:* Sexuality at Mid-life and beyond
• Hysterectomy is a safe and effective means of sterilization for a woman who does not want any more children.	*Part 3:* Hysterectomy and Surgical Menopause
• All women have an equal chance of breaking bones due to osteoporosis after menopause.	*Part 2:* Osteoporosis
• If you have a positive attitude and stay active, you will sail through your menopause.	*Part 2:* Introduction

13

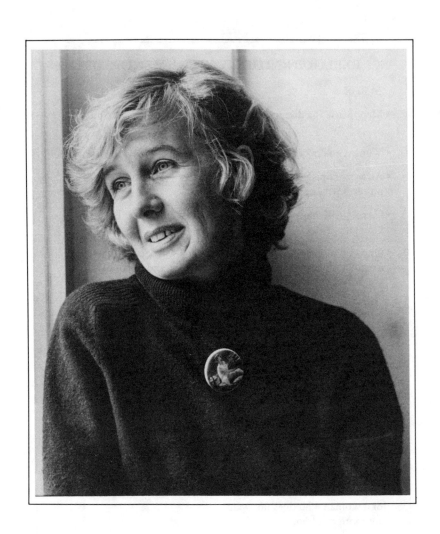

PART ONE

THE TIME OF YOUR LIFE

Menopause is the end of menstruation. It is a single event which marks the end of the fertile period of your life that began with puberty. Menopause is an experience of mid-life just as teething is part of childhood and puberty is part of adolescence. Our experiences of these biological events are shaped by interactions between the events themselves and other things happening in our lives.

Much of this book focuses on understanding the process of menopause in all its aspects. This section is devoted to the context in which menopause occurs — both the common experiences of mid-life women and the larger social and political issues.

THE MID-LIFE CONTEXT

Each stage in a person's life brings with it new issues to face, tasks to accomplish, psychological and biological changes to experience. As we live though each stage, we learn things and gain skills which we can use in the future.

15

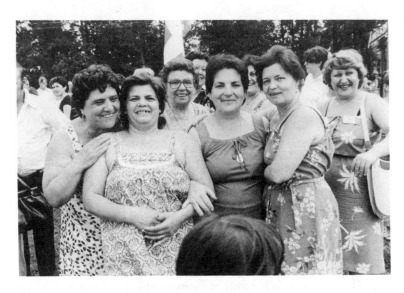

"I think there is an autumn. From an existential point of view, there is the period of life where things are sad. You go through that period saying goodbye to certain things and you mourn something. I think it is normal. And in the years that follow you take into account that it is the other side of life. And I think it must also be sad for men. It's not because you are a woman and your physiological function stops."

Mid-life is a period of 15 to 20 years at the midway point of adulthood, between the ages of about 40 to 60. It is not an empty space between raising children and old age, but a stage of life full of its own joys and problems. As with other mid-points, it offers a chance to stop and take stock, this time with the benefit of hindsight and greater awareness. For some, mid-life is a time of introspection, when we review who we are, where we have been and where we want to go. We may acknowledge achievements, confront failures, resolve difficulties and accept that we are getting older. This mid-life review can provide insights into our lives and encourage the setting of new goals for our work and leisure as we look ahead to the future.

Often those goals centre around having more free time for ourselves. As our focus shifts from meeting others' needs to meeting our own, we may find ourselves having more free time than we want. We may need to seek out new activities and renew friendships. We may increase our work hours or choose to return to the work force. Our families and friends may not be ready to change with us. If they do not want to relinquish some of our attention or if they cannot support us through any stressful times, this period can become one of anger and conflict.

Most of us confront the aging process at this stage in our lives. Our awareness of the passage of time may be heightened by the changes in our bodies, by watching our parents grow older or our children become adults. Menopause does not herald the coming of old age, but contributes to our awareness of aging because it symbolizes the end of one life-cycle phase and the start of a new one.

"There were some elements of sadness. Even though I no longer realistically wanted children I did feel a sort of pang. Of course I won't miss my periods per se — who would — but the idea of them. It's such a miracle really. Conception and no longer conceiving, well it is the end of a stage."

Mid-life brings with it the end of our reproductive capacity. Those who had a difficult time with menstruation or struggled with imperfect birth control methods may welcome the end of these worries. Or we may take bittersweet note of

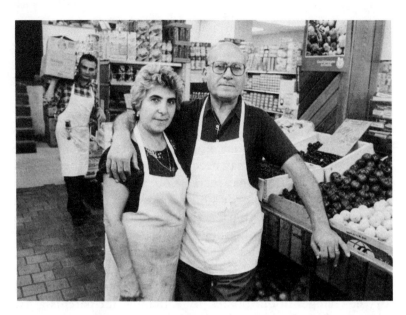

the passing of this era. For those among us who thought about one more child but kept waiting for the right moment, menopause brings the realization that the moment will never come. If we did not have children, whether or not by choice, we must face the fact that we will remain childless.

At mid-life, many of us with children are either living with adolescents or watching our children leave home. Much has been said of the empty-nest syndrome; we often feel sad when our offspring move on. Yet more and more, women describe a sense of relief and joy at having time for themselves, rediscovering old interests and developing new ones. The children's departure leaves us face to face with our partner again, without the common goal of childrearing. Some women find this relationship improves once the stresses of living with adolescent and adult children are removed. Others discover that they and their partner have grown in different directions, and the relationship crumbles.

Those of us who worked at home raising our children may

respond differently to the children's departure than those who also worked outside the home. If caring for children and family was our full-time work, then the children's departure is analogous to retirement, and may spark the same kind of identity crisis. Although the novelty of having time to think about ourselves can be exciting, choosing a new line of work after so many years can be very stressful.

❖

"We should mention that when your own daughter begins to do some of the exciting things that you have done in the past and is doing them very well at a time when you are doing nothing, there is a trauma."

❖

"As I am getting older I seem to be enjoying life more. I loved being a mother, but I put in my time and I'm really ready to let that nurturing go and to start looking after me."

❖

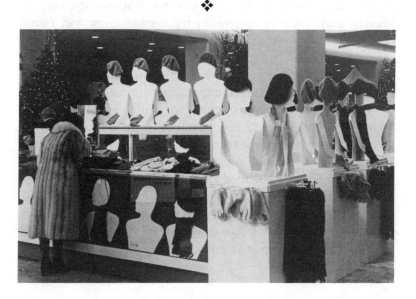

For those in the paid work force, our children's departure does not signal retirement. In fact, as working women at mid-life, whether or not we have children, we are at the peak of our work experience. This may be a period of great satisfaction and striving to attain goals at work. It can also be a time of hard work and stress. Many women talk about the stresses and adjustments required by a new reality — the revolving door syndrome — where adult children move home again after they lose their jobs or end their marriages or just need help to make ends meet.

Family responsibilities do not end after the children have left home; they are part of our lives even if we never had children. At mid-life, we are still the primary caregivers for our families, including our partner, aging parents and in-laws. Although some men are taking a more active role in childcare, care of aging parents still falls primarily on women's shoulders. We make doctors' appointments and then take care of the chauffeuring to those appointments. We monitor the emotional well-being of our family, cook, shop and sometimes provide full-time nursing care at home. Without the help of professional resources provided by homemakers and home care nurses, this job can be a major source of physical and emotional strain. The growing emphasis on home care over institutional care has forced us to take on more of this role, sometimes at great financial expense, and even at the expense of our paid jobs. In most cases we willingly and lovingly provide this care to our families. Yet so little recognition is given to this work that it seems almost invisible. The services and resources that could permit us to take care of our families without being overwhelmed are often unavailable.

Our mid-life experiences are unique to each of us. The quality of our lives is determined by such a wide range of factors — from genes to economics to just plain luck — that it is impossible to imagine any two of us with exactly the same mid-life experience. Still, there are some common themes in women's lives.

THE POLITICS OF MENOPAUSE

Beyond the personal context, the experience of menopause is profoundly affected by social factors. Our society's views on women, aging, sexuality and reproduction all play a part in the development of our own attitudes towards menopause and the commonly held myths that surround it. Many historical, social, cultural and medical factors have led to the development of these myths and attitudes. We need to understand where the stereotypes of menopausal women come from. Then we can begin to replace these stereotypes with a more accurate, individualized understanding of the experience of menopause.

Historical Factors
At the turn of the century, when the average life expectancy of women was about 55, menopause coincided with a woman's final years. In North America today, the average age at menopause is 50, and life expectancy is 79. Most of us can expect to live about thirty years after menopause. Yet in spite of the radically different life expectancies of the 1990s menopause continues to be seen by many as the first sign of old age. This view also results from the belief that our primary function is reproduction. Despite widespread use of birth control and sterilization, which mean the end of reproduction for many women long before menopause, this attitude persists. When reproducing is no longer possible, the stereotype tells us our meaningful life is considered over — but in reality we continue to live active lives for decades.

Our reproductive organs have long been considered the source of many health problems. In the nineteenth century, medicine developed the concept of "hysteria," or the wandering womb, which travelled through a woman's body leaving dramatic symptoms in its wake. Physical activity, sexual arousal, dancing, working and even thinking were thought to drain energy from the reproductive organs, making us sick. Our ovaries in particular were linked to mental health; in the late nineteenth century, thousands of women had their ovaries removed to treat such "mental illnesses" as nymphomania (excessive interest in sex), anti-social behaviour and depression.

This perspective has changed and evolved over the years, but has not entirely disappeared. On the one hand, our hormones and reproductive organs are still seen as a source of problems; on the other hand these same problems are considered imaginary. Difficulties ranging from painful periods to morning sickness are often treated as symptoms of our discomfort with our feminine or maternal identity rather than as real physical problems. Similarly, menopausal problems are seen by some as a reflection of our inability to let go of our reproductive function and face the inevitable aging process.

Social and Cultural Factors

Our attitudes and actions are all influenced by the rules and expectations of the society in which we live. Society's norms govern our behaviour, our understanding of situations and the content of our shared beliefs.

In our society many norms reflect what is usual for men. For example, our biology, especially reproductive biology, is perceived as outside the norm. Because the steady level of hormones which men experience is considered the norm, our fluctuating hormone levels have been blamed for our supposed irrationality and instability, and have been used as an excuse for barring us from positions of power and responsibility. The irony is that once our hormone levels are no longer cyclic — after menopause — we are considered estrogen-deprived, and therefore still abnormal.

22

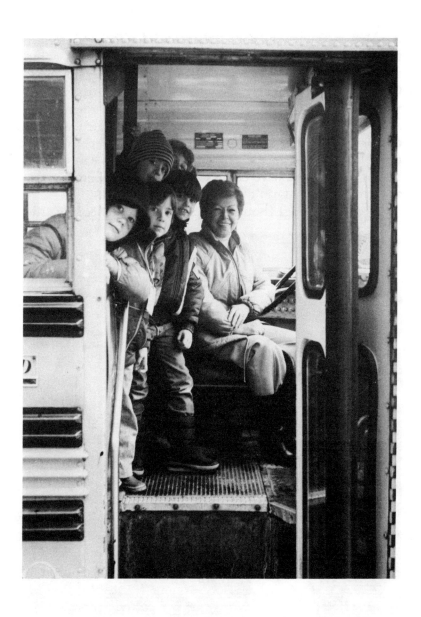

Many attitudes and approaches toward menopause reflect the "fast-food" nature of our modern society. We have come to expect easy solutions, and pills to make troubles go away. Often people feel vaguely dissatisfied leaving a doctor's office without a prescription, even if the doctor gave them good advice about diet and exercise. Some feel frustrated when a doctor cannot offer a fast cure. This "fast food" culture extends beyond the doctor's office. We don't take care of our bodies because we have come to believe that science can fix anything, and what can't be fixed can be replaced.

People's feelings about menopause are influenced by atti-

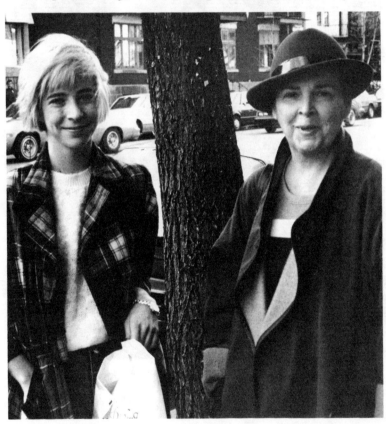

tudes towards aging. Ageism is prejudice or discrimination against a person based on age. Older people are seen as less competent than the young, and their bodies seen as unattractive. Although our preoccupation with youth affects both sexes, women are particularly vulnerable to ageism. Middle-aged men, but not their female counterparts, are portrayed as distinguished, wise and still in their prime.

Attitudes linking menopause and aging with many negative characteristics have traditionally forced women to hide their experience from those around them, preventing them from comparing experiences and sharing solutions. In recent years, this has begun to change.

The women's movement, and particularly the women's health movement, have influenced how we approach menopause. The early focus of these movements was on birth control, abortion and childbirth — issues of younger women. Over the years, as we have grown older, the focus has extended to include issues of mid-life and old age. Greater access to information, an increased openness to discussing menopause, and critical feminist analysis of the issues are some of the benefits we have gained from this larger focus.

Medical Factors

Women are the main users of the health care system in North America. From the time our periods begin, we see doctors and use hospitals more frequently than men. This high rate of contact with the system is linked to our reproductive organs. We require birth control, give birth to babies, have Pap smears and take hormone replacement therapy. Though these visits usually take place when we are well, we are cared for by doctors who are trained by and for a system that focuses on illness. As a result, our normal life events such as childbirth and menopause are treated as illnesses. Although these events do have an impact on our health and can sometimes cause illness, they are in themselves normal and healthy.

25

The medical treatment — and sometimes overtreatment — of normal life events is called "medicalization". It profoundly affects many aspects of the menopause experience. For example, medical books that describe menopause as a "deficiency syndrome" or "ovarian failure" teach doctors, and through them us, their patients, that menopause is a disease in which something is lost or has gone awry. Through the process of medicalization, this female rite of passage has been defined as an illness.

Defining menopause as illness has two effects. First, doctors, as the unchallenged experts on illness, have become the experts on menopause. What we as "ordinary" women know is considered less significant than what the "experts" have to say. Second, once a series of events is labelled as illness, it is logical to look for a cure — something that will remedy the deficiency or make the patient "better". For menopausal women, this means hormone replacement. All the changes associated with menopause, from the most minor to the totally incapacitating, are seen as treatable conditions under the model of menopause as disease.

Drug companies that manufacture chemical treatments for menopause symptoms also have a significant role in moulding opinions about menopause and hormone replacement therapy. For years their notorious advertisements in medical journals depicted menopausal women as falling apart. Their pictures portrayed women spoiling the lives of family, friends, employers and in one particularly insulting ad, even the local bus driver. In response to protest and pressure on the drug companies, these ads have recently become more subtle. Menopausal women are now portrayed as having lost something which must be replaced.

Drug companies influence the practice of medicine in other ways as well, by sponsoring conferences, funding research, and providing perks for doctors. For example, Dr. Robert Wilson, a gynecologist and the author of *Feminine*

Forever, a book published in 1966 and widely read for many years, was one of the first proponents of the theory of menopause as a disease. He called it a state of "living decay" in which we lose our womanhood and our good health. His solution, proposed in many respected professional journals, was to treat us with hormones from puberty to death. Most women who read his book did not know that his research was funded by a drug company that produced and sold estrogen.

The medicalization of menopause has potential economic benefits for doctors. The payment system of "fee for service" creates an incentive for frequent medical visits.

Fear of lawsuits from women who experience side effects from hormone therapy has begun to affect the way doctors treat menopausal women. Some try to protect themselves against lawsuits by prescribing more tests, even if they are expensive, uncomfortable or potentially dangerous. Some have opted for a different strategy, encouraging the woman's participation in the decision-making process so that the decision to take the hormones is essentially her own.

Research Factors

The knowledge and practice of professionals within the health care system is based on research which has been accumulating over many years. Good professionals continue to read about the areas in which they work so that their understanding and decisions are based on the most up-to-date knowledge available. However, biased research may lead to faulty knowledge and practice.

Many qualified researchers suggest that research biases have indeed had an impact on our knowledge about menopause. For example, studies about many changes happening around menopause have traditionally been done on those women most convenient to study — those who consult doctors. This is called a clinical sample, because the people studied are found in a clinical setting. Findings from clinical samples

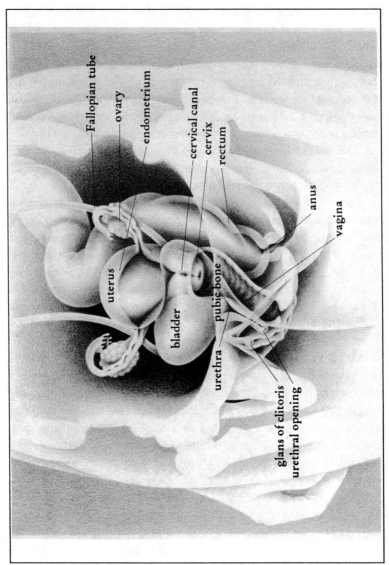

Fallopian tube
ovary
endometrium
cervical canal
cervix
rectum
anus
vagina
uterus
bladder
pubic bone
urethra
glans of clitoris
urethral opening

FEMALE SEXUAL AND REPRODUCTIVE ORGANS

can be biased because the people interviewed tend to have problems or they wouldn't be at the doctor's office. When these findings are used to make statements about the general population, we often get an unrealistic view of how women are experiencing menopause.

How research questions are chosen is also relevant to menopause. Choices are influenced by the personal interest of the researchers and the priorities of funding agencies, both of which have a high proportion of men. Also, the questions which are researched tend to reflect the philosophy or framework of the researchers, so that much of the medical research on menopause reflects the medical model of menopause as a deficiency syndrome. As a result there are few if any studies of the effectiveness of natural remedies for menopausal symptoms, but lots of research on hormone replacement.

A final concern is an emphasis on research which generates quantitative results, for example, the number of women who get hot flashes. There is much less research that looks at women's *experiences* of hot flashes.

As women, our biology is not a medical problem, but an interesting, intricate and normal part of us. We have the judgment and competence to understand what is happening to our bodies and to make decisions about our health.

To make informed choices we need more information, as well as an open and accepting environment in which to discuss the issues. We need to be aware of alternatives to traditional medical and social ways of dealing with menopause, and we need access to them. We also need traditional medicine to change — to become more responsive to our needs and to us as individuals. This requires changes in priorities of clinicians, researchers and funding agencies. And we, as mid-life women, must step forward to define and defend our interests.

HORMONE SOURCES

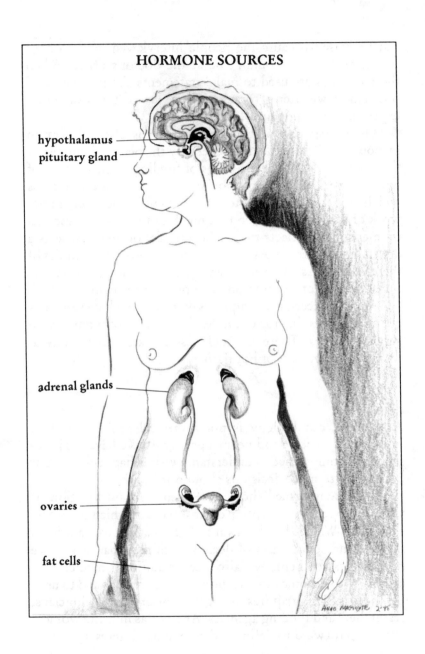

hypothalamus

pituitary gland

adrenal glands

ovaries

fat cells

HORMONE FEEDBACK SYSTEM

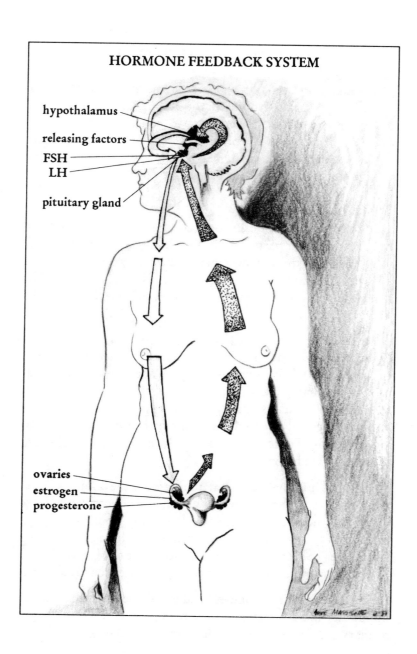

hypothalamus

releasing factors

FSH

LH

pituitary gland

ovaries
estrogen
progesterone

THE BIOLOGICAL PROCESS

Menopause, or the end of menstruation, is the result of changes in the levels of sex hormones in the blood. Although you need not become a hormone specialist to cope with menopause, some familiarity with the hormones involved in the menstrual cycle makes it easier to understand the physical and emotional changes that many of us experience.

Sex Hormones

A hormone is a chemical produced in an organ or gland and carried to another part of the body via the bloodstream. There it acts as a chemical messenger, stimulating that body part, known as the target organ, to carry out its usual function. The hormones which affect the menstrual cycle, and therefore, the process of menopause, are produced in four parts of our bodies.

Hypothalamus. This part of the brain plays a major role in coordinating bodily functions such as appetite and temperature control. It is also involved in regulating psychological states and in the menstrual cycle. The hypothalamus produces hormones (called releasing factors) which stimulate the pituitary to release Follicle Stimulating Hormone and Luteinizing Hormone (see below).

Pituitary. This small gland at the base of the brain is often referred to as the body's master gland; it produces a very large number of hormones which regulate many bodily functions including growth and reproduction. Follicle Stimulating Hormone (FSH) and Luteinizing Hormone (LH) are the two pituitary hormones which help to regulate the menstrual cycle.

Ovary. These two almond-shaped glands lie on either side of the uterus and are attached to it by a ligament. They are the primary source of the hormones estrogen and progesterone in

32

women until menopause. At birth, the ovaries contain imma-
ture egg sacs (follicles). Beginning at puberty, several eggs
mature each month, and one is released in a process called
ovulation.

Adrenal glands. These glands, situated on top of the kidneys,
are best known for the adrenaline they produce in stressful
situations. They release many other hormones including estrogen and testosterone. Another adrenal hormone is con-
verted in body fat into a form of estrogen called estrone.

There are five main hormones which regulate the menstrual
cycle from puberty to menopause:

FSH (Follicle Stimulating Hormone) is produced by the pituitary gland and stimulates the ovary to produce estrogen. FSH
also promotes the growth of several egg-containing follicles,
one of which ruptures to release an egg at ovulation. In the
years just before menopause and for a number of years after,
FSH levels in the blood are very high.

LH (Luteinizing Hormone) produced in the pituitary also
affects the ovary. LH is necessary for the follicle to burst open
at ovulation. The ruptured follicle then transforms into a
hormone-secreting organ called the corpus luteum, which
produces the hormone progesterone. As with FSH, LH levels
are high in the years surrounding menopause.

Estrogen, produced primarily in the ovaries throughout the
reproductive years, has many target organs: it is important for
the development of the follicles; it stimulates the endometrium
(lining of the uterus) to develop and thicken each month; and
it is necessary for ovulation. It also stimulates the mucous
membranes of the vagina, keeping them elastic and well lubricated, and protects against the loss of bone density which can
lead to osteoporosis (see page 70). After menopause the ovaries continue to produce estrogen, but in smaller quantities.

Progesterone is produced by the corpus luteum (ruptured follicle) during the reproductive years. It is important for the development of the uterine lining. After menopause small quantities of progesterone are produced by the adrenal glands.

Androgens are often referred to as male hormones but are produced by both sexes. In women, the best known of the androgens, testosterone, is produced by the ovaries and the adrenal glands. Researchers are studying the influence of androgens on sex drive. In large amounts androgens increase

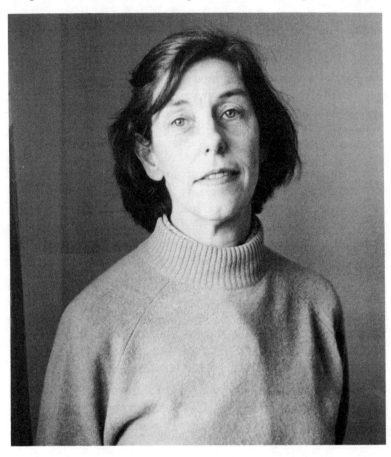

body hair and muscle mass, and lower the pitch of a person's voice.

The hormones which control the menstrual cycle are interrelated. Together they make up a system known as the *hypothalamic-pituitary-ovarian axis*. The diagrams on pages 30/31 show how these hormones act in relation to each other. The role of the axis is to prepare our bodies each month for conception and pregnancy. It does this by regulating the amounts of estrogen and progesterone circulating in our bloodstream.

The axis is based on a negative feedback system, much like the thermostat of a furnace. When a sensor in the thermostat cools off, the furnace turns on. Similarly, low estrogen and progesterone levels in the bloodstream trigger the hypothalamus to secrete releasing factors. A chain reaction occurs: the releasing factors stimulate the pituitary to release FSH (Follicle Stimulating Hormone) and LH (Luteinizing Hormone). These two hormones cause the ovaries to produce estrogen and progesterone which stimulate ovulation.

Just as high temperatures shut off the furnace, the high levels of estrogen and progesterone in the blood trigger a decrease in the production of the hypothalamic and pituitary hormones. As the releasing factors decrease, so do FSH and LH, triggering a reduction in estrogen and progesterone until the levels are so low that the whole system starts up again.

THE STAGES OF MENOPAUSE

Just as puberty and the onset of fertility were marked not only by your first period, but by a host of other changes (breast growth, pubic hair, etc.), menopause brings both your last period and other body changes as well. In both cases, many of the changes occur due to varying levels of sex hormones. Other aspects of the experience may be more linked to social expectations and cultural factors.

As with puberty, it takes a few years for all of the adjustments to be made and for a new hormonal balance to be reached. When we talk about menopause we are usually referring to this more extended period rather than to the last menstruation.

There has been a language problem with regard to menopause. Although menopause officially refers to a single event — the end of menstruation, people have used it to mean the years surrounding that event. They may say "I'm going through my menopause" for a period of months or even years. We have chosen the following definitions for the stages of the menopausal transition, but you will sometimes see the same terms defined differently.

Pre-Menopause: the time of greatest hormone fluctuation during the later reproductive years, when periods become irregular, and other changes may begin to occur.

The early changes of pre-menopause are triggered by one simple alteration in the hormonal feedback system which controls the menstrual cycle (see page 31). Your ovaries become less responsive to the stimulation of FSH released by the pituitary. The precise reason for this is unknown, but it is probably linked to the decreasing number of egg follicles on the ovary. A baby girl is born with approximately 2 million follicles in her ovaries. Most of them disappear. By puberty only about 250,000 remain. More follicles are used up during each menstrual cycle. By pre-menopause, the few remaining follicles are probably the least responsive to FSH.

With fewer active follicles, your ovaries produce less estrogen. This sets off the expected response. The pituitary produces more FSH trying to increase the level of estrogen in the blood. Follicles begin to mature but they secrete little estrogen. When none of the follicles matures enough to release

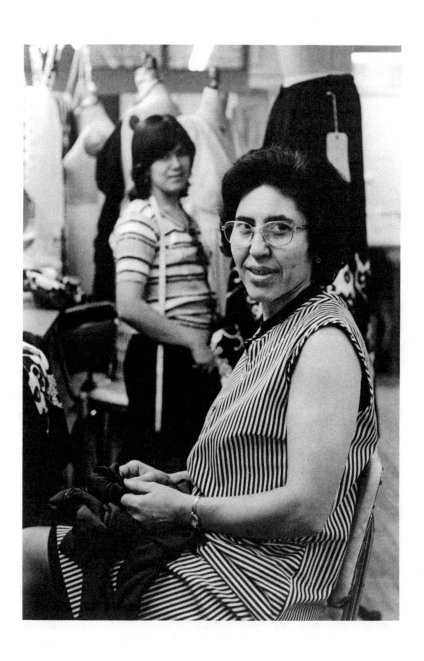

an egg there is no ovulation (called an anovulatory cycle). In an anovulatory cycle no corpus luteum (the remnant of the ruptured follicle) is formed and therefore no progesterone is secreted. The level of LH then rises in the blood, as the pituitary tries to stimulate progesterone production.

High FSH and LH levels are the hallmark of the pre- and post-menopausal periods. We cannot feel these elevated hormone levels. They can only be detected by blood tests.

Early in pre-menopause, the hormonal feedback system is working, but your cycle may be a bit shorter or longer than when you were younger. Later during pre-menopause, you may experience anovulatory cycles some months, while other months the orderly events of the menstrual cycle occur without disruption. This variability has a number of consequences. You are less fertile than you were before, and you may experience changes in your cycle length and amount of flow. Many women begin to have hot flashes in the pre-menopause.

Menopause: the end of menstruation; defined after the fact, that is, once 12 months have gone by without a period.

Eventually your ovaries stop responding to FSH no matter how high the levels get. Then there is no ovulation. Nor is enough estrogen produced to build up the lining of your uterus (endometrium). With nothing to shed you stop having periods. This is menopause.

Menopause can happen in three ways: 1) periods can remain regular and then stop suddenly; 2) they can change in a regular pattern (e.g. cycle gets longer or shorter) and eventually stop; or 3) they can fluctuate in an irregular pattern until they stop. The third pattern is the most common.

Regardless of your pattern, it is only possible to know after the fact — a year later — that a particular period was your last one. This can be disconcerting if you are still using birth control and aren't sure if it is safe to stop yet. It may also be frustrating if you would like to know whether you have passed through your menopause.

Women who have had a hysterectomy but still have their ovaries cannot depend on the absence of periods to determine when they have had their menopause.

Post-Menopause: the several years after the end of menstruation during which the body completes its adaptation to its new hormonal state.

After the last period, your ovaries continue to produce estrogen in smaller quantities, decreasing slowly and erratically over the years. Your body has other sources of estrogen which produce a larger proportion of the hormones once the role of the ovaries diminishes. The adrenal glands, situated on top of each kidney, produce estrogen as well as other chemicals which are turned into estrogen in the body's fat cells.

The amount of estrogen that circulates in the blood after menopause varies from woman to woman, and depends on a number of factors. Heavier women tend to have more estrogen since body fat is one of the sites where the hormone is produced. This explains why thinner women often have more difficulty with some aspects of menopause, particularly osteoporosis (see page 76).

Women who have a surgical menopause (have their ovaries removed before they go through menopause) have lower levels of estrogen and other ovarian hormones such as testosterone. The drop in hormone levels takes place suddenly at the time of surgery, and symptoms are often more severe as a result.

Women who have their ovaries removed after they have gone through menopause will have a less dramatic drop in estrogen because their estrogen levels will already be decreasing. However they will have lower testosterone levels than other women their age who still have their ovaries.

Peri-Menopause refers to the years surrounding the event of menopause. It includes the late pre-menopause and the early post-menopause.

Surgical Menopause is menopause brought on by the surgical removal of a woman's ovaries or by radiation treatment. If you have not already gone through a natural menopause when you have your surgery or treatment, you will go through immediate menopause at that time, and you will skip the pre- and peri-menopausal stages.

Later On

At a certain point we stop orienting ourselves around our menopause. Our hormone levels stabilize and we can consider ourselves as having passed through that stage in our lives. Although our bodies continue to change, these are no longer

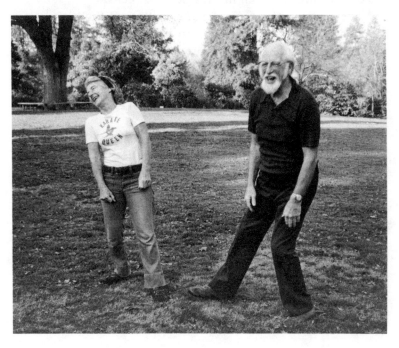

menopausal changes, but rather the general effects of aging that touch us all, women and men alike.

Many women talk about this time of their lives in very positive terms. They feel well both physically and emotionally. They may experience an upswing of energy, something that anthropologist Margaret Mead aptly called post-menopausal zest!

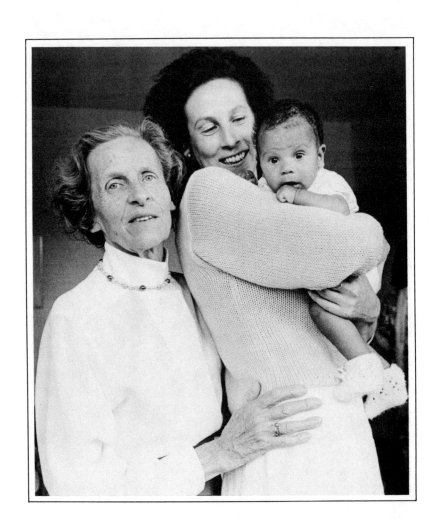

PART TWO

CHANGES FROM A TO Z

Menopause is a very individual experience, influenced by a myriad of personal factors including general health, reproductive history and genetic background. Cultural and social factors, though less completely understood, also have an important impact. We each have our own menopause. Some of us experience problems and some sail through. Later in life, some of us feel the effects of low estrogen levels, while others do not. It is difficult to predict what any given woman will experience. A positive attitude and a bit of perspective always help, but many other factors also influence whether menopause will be easy or difficult.

Physical and emotional changes which can occur during and after menopause may be temporary or long term. As you go through menopause, you may experience a few of them or none at all.

This part of the book is about the changes that menopause brings with it, and can be used in different ways. You can look up specific changes you are experiencing for information on why they are happening and what you can do about them. Or you can read right through to get an overall picture. You will

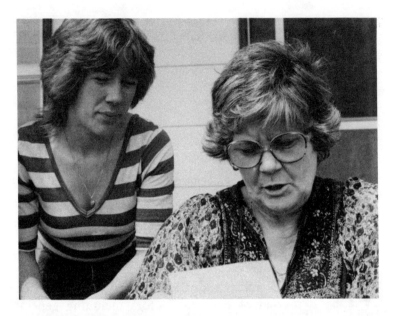

not only find information about your own menopause, but will gain insight into other women's experiences as well.

The most commonly studied and talked about changes associated with menopause are menstrual cycle and vaginal changes, hot flashes and osteoporosis. In this book we refer to them as "the big four". They are much easier to account for than the other things women experience around menopause because they can be linked directly to hormones.

MENSTRUAL CYCLE CHANGES

"There was no irregularity until close to the end — I'd say during the last two years that I menstruated. Then there were two 6 month periods without one. I'd just figure that's it, it is over, and then I would get a period. Then not another one for 6 months again."

What Are They?

Changes in the menstrual cycle are often our first sign that menopause is approaching. They may be sudden and significant, or so gradual that we hardly notice them. Periods may be very different from what they once were. Menstrual-cycle changes can affect cycle length and the amount of menstrual flow.

"When I was 37 my periods became irregular. Sometimes I had it and sometimes not. The worst part of it was that when I had it, it was almost like labour pains. I had to be taken to the hospital several times. This went on for 3 or 4 months and then I had the first D&C."

Cycle Length: In the years before menopause you may find your periods coming more or less frequently, and you may at times skip periods entirely. Sometimes your regular menstrual pattern returns for a few months, and then the changes will recur. Eventually your periods stop completely.

"My periods became awfully erratic and I would miss some completely. I had some heavy periods around that time as well. But I was expecting it, so the element of surprise was entirely missing. Also, I had always been a bit pre-menstrual, you know headachy and cranky a bit. And that sort of got more intense."

Most women we spoke with expected some changes in their periods before menopause and did not find they caused much anxiety. However these changes can cause some practical concerns. For example women who could predict the start of their periods almost to the minute may have to join their less "regular" sisters in carrying around pads or tampons for unexpected bleeding. Also, although you are less fertile at this time, pregnancy is still a possibility, and very irregular periods can lead to pregnancy scares.

Menstrual Flow. In the years before menopause your menstrual flow may increase, decrease or stay the same. Your periods may range from short and scanty to long and heavy.

Two kinds of heavy bleeding can occur. Each may require medical attention, but for different reasons. The first is flooding, where the flow may be so heavy that it is impossible to stay dry for more than a few minutes. Heavy bleeding which is unmanageable may require a doctor's help to bring under control. Pre-menopausal flooding is not a sign of cancer or serious disease, but can be very frightening because we tend to associate heavy bleeding with life-threatening situations. Unmanageable bleeding leaves you feeling out of control. It can be very disruptive, making work and normal daily activities difficult to carry out.

The second type of heavy flow is repeated heavy bleeding. Although the actual amount of blood loss with each period may not be as great, the fact that it recurs month after month often leads to chronic anemia. Very heavy flow should be reported to the doctor who will do a blood test to check for anemia.

Anemia is a decrease in hemoglobin, the iron-containing molecules in the blood which carry oxygen. It can result from any kind of heavy bleeding. The symptoms of anemia, including fatigue, paleness and weakness are not always obvious, so if you have been having heavy periods, your hemoglobin should be checked (by blood test).

Breakthrough Bleeding. This term refers to irregular bleeding between periods. It can be heavy or light, red or brown. Around menopause, breakthrough bleeding is often related to

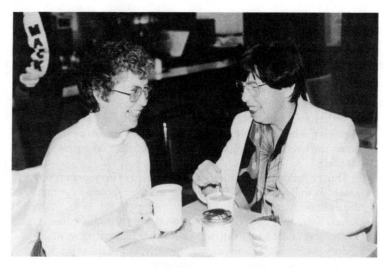

hormonal factors that cause irregular shedding of the endometrial lining. There can be other causes as well, including vaginal or cervical problems. Some post-menopausal women experience bleeding after intercourse due to irritation of fragile vaginal tissue which is not sufficiently lubricated during intercourse.

Bleeding between periods or any bleeding in women who are no longer having periods can be a sign of cancer of the reproductive organs, and should be reported to a doctor.

Who Gets Them?

Most women experience some menstrual cycle changes during the years surrounding menopause. Although there are some whose periods stop suddenly, most go through a few months or even years of variability before that last period. Women with endometrial overgrowth (hyperplasia) and those who take estrogen therapy alone are more likely to have abnormal cycle changes.

CAUSES OF MENSTRUAL CYCLE CHANGES48

During the reproductive years, the sex hormones control ovulation (release of an egg) and menstruation. FSH, LH and estrogen cause ovulation. Estrogen stimulates the growth of the uterine lining. Progesterone, produced by the ruptured follicle (corpus luteum), controls the further growth of the lining. When pregnancy does not occur, the level of estrogen and progesterone falls, causing menstrual bleeding.

During the pre-menopause, the production of hormones is no longer so well balanced. The following situations account for the different menstrual cycle changes:

1. **Less Estrogen:** The aging follicles on the ovary produce less estrogen. A decrease in estrogen affects the endometrium which does not thicken as usual during the early part of the cycle. With less lining to be shed, periods are scantier.

2. **Less Progesterone:** After ovulation the corpus luteum on the ovary may produce less progesterone. When levels of this hormone drop earlier in the cycle, an earlier menstruation is triggered and the cycle will be shorter.

3. **Extended Progesterone Effect:** Sometimes the corpus luteum does not shrink in the usual way after ovulation (release of the egg at mid-cycle). The persistence of progesterone causes the endometrium to build up past the point in the cycle where it would normally be shed. However, without enough progesterone to completely prevent endometrial breakdown, women experience erratic bleeding over an extended time, continuing into the next cycle (breakthrough bleeding).

4. **Lack of Ovulation:** Periodically ovulation does not take place during a cycle. This can affect both cycle length and amount of flow. Without ovulation, estrogen stimulates the development of the endometrium, but the corpus luteum does not form and progesterone is not produced. The endometrium becomes overgrown, extremely dense and fragile. The woman's period will be late because there is no progesterone drop-off to stimulate a normal menstruation. When it does come the flow is usually heavier and longer, and often is accompanied by cramps. Anovulatory cycles may also cause breakthrough bleeding if only parts of the endometrium break down at different times.

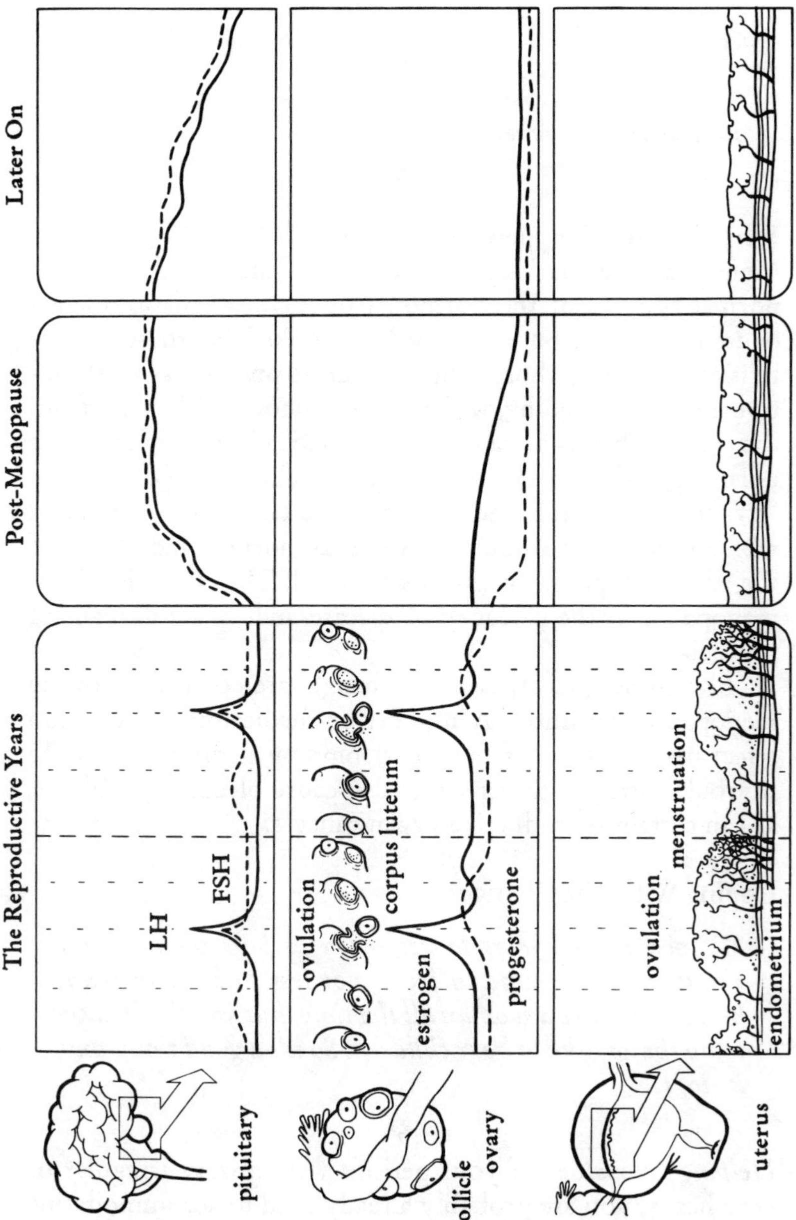

MENSTRUAL CYCLE CHANGES

The Reproductive Years

Post-Menopause

Later On

pituitary

LH

FSH

follicle

ovary

ovulation

corpus luteum

estrogen

progesterone

uterus

ovulation

menstruation

endometrium

49

❖

*"I went on (menstruating) until I was 44. Then it stopped
just like that! I never saw it again."*

❖

Why Do They Happen?

Menstrual irregularities in both cycle length and flow are
normal because of the hormonal fluctuations of pre-menopause (see inset). But most medical books label these irregularities as well as those which occur at puberty as dysfunctional uterine bleeding, which means abnormal bleeding from
the uterus. This is an example of the medicalization of women's
normal physiological processes. By labeling these changes as
"dysfunctional", the medical profession defines the cycles of a
woman in her reproductive years as normal and those of
the peri-menopausal years as abnormal. This attitude places
menopause in the category of disease and in the domain of
physicians.

Sometimes menstrual cycle changes are not a result of the
menopause transition. A number of medical conditions can
affect periods. One of the most common is problems of the
thyroid. Estrogen therapy can also cause bleeding problems,
as can certain reproductive-organ cancers.

Coping With The Changes

*"It took me 13 years to get ready to be a woman and
about the same time to feel... not less to be a woman,
because you are a woman all the time, but you don't have
to do things, like to bear children. So it's a good thing that
it stops."*

Helping Ourselves. If your periods were always irregular or
very heavy, you are probably already used to accommodating
yourself to erratic periods, and these changes may be no more

MENSTRUAL CHART

MARCH

DATE	7	8	9	10	11	12	13	14	15	16	17	18	19	20	21	22	23	24	25	26	27	28	29	30	31
Bleeding	X	X	X	X	X	X	X	X					X	X									X	X	X
Day of cycle	1	2	3	4	5	6	7	8	9	10	11	12	13	14	15	16	17	18	19	20	21	22	1	2	3
*Amount of bleeding	H	H	H	H	M	M	M	M					L	L									H	H	M
Other	cramps breast pain	cramps clots																			sad irritable	irritable cramps clots	sad irritable cramps cramps		
Sexual intercourse							X			X	X							X							

APRIL

DATE	1	2	3	4	5	6	7	8	9	10	11	12	13	14	15	16	17	18	19	20	21	22	23	24	25
Bleeding	X	X	X	X																					X
Day of cycle	4	5	6	7	8	9	10	11	12	13	14	15	16	17	18	19	20	21	22	23	24	25	26	27	1
*Amount of bleeding	M	M	L	L																					L
Other									vaginal discharge	cramps											bloated irritable	bloated irritable	cramps	cramps	
Sexual intercourse				X	X								X												

* F = flooding   M = moderate
  H = heavy   L = light

51

than a minor annoyance. If your periods were more predictable, these changes will require more of an adjustment.

A first step in coping with menstrual cycle changes is to get a clear picture of what is actually happening by keeping track of your periods. Try setting up a menstrual chart: record the date your period began, the amount of flow and any bleeding in between. The length of the menstrual cycle is determined by counting from the first day of one period to the first day of the next. If the second period starts on the 32nd day, then the cycle length for that month is 31 days.

A menstrual chart gives you an instant history of your peri-menopause. It is useful when consulting the doctor. A chart helps you to figure out if you could be pregnant when

---

IRON CONTENT OF SOME FOODS

	AMOUNT	IRON*
pork liver	90 g (3 oz)	26.1 mg
seaweed (dried)	100 g (3.3 oz)	10-17 mg
prune juice	250 ml (1 cup)	11 mg
dried apricots	250 ml (1 cup)	8.6 mg
beef liver	90 g (3 oz)	8 mg
chicken liver	90 g (3 oz)	7.7 mg
raisins	250 ml (1 cup)	6.1 mg
clams	90 g (3 oz)	5.5 mg
oysters (raw)	90 g (3 oz)	5.1 mg
spinach (cooked)	250 ml (1 cup)	4.2 mg
almonds	125 ml (1/2 cup)	4 mg
lentils (cooked)	250 ml (1 cup)	3.3 mg
blackstrap molasses	1 tbsp	3.2 mg
peas (cooked)	250 ml (1 cup)	3.0 mg
ground beef (broiled)	90 g (3 oz)	2.9 mg

*Figures taken from Health and Welfare Canada, Nutrient Value of Some Common Foods.

The recommended intake of iron per day for women still menstruating is 14 mg. Once menopause is over, the requirements drop to 7 mg/day.

your periods are irregular, and lets you know when you have officially had your menopause, i.e. when 12 months have passed since your last period.

Some women deal with the uncertainty of irregular periods by having occasional pregnancy tests. Around menopause, pregnancy tests can be less reliable since high levels of pituitary hormones (FSH and LH) can be mistaken for the hormones of pregnancy.

Keep an eye out for early signs of pregnancy (breast tenderness, fatigue, nausea, etc.). Natural birth control methods which monitor body temperature, cervical secretions and other signs of ovulation are more complicated to use for birth control during the menopausal transition, but could alert you early on to the possibility of pregnancy. Birth control methods for the pre-menopausal woman are discussed in the section about sexuality (page 158).

Unlike some of the milder changes, heavy bleeding and flooding can create stress and disruption in your life. You will likely look for specific ways to control the bleeding.

One way to take care of yourself if you have heavy periods is to prevent anemia by increasing the amount of iron in your diet. The chart on page 52 lists foods which are high in iron. Iron supplements can also be useful, especially if you are already anemic.

The most effective form of iron supplement is ferrous iron which is the most easily absorbed from the intestines. Though iron is absorbed best when taken on an empty stomach, it can cause side effects like nausea, diarrhea or constipation. (If you have problems, take it with meals.) Vitamin C increases the absorption of iron, so try taking it with a glass of orange juice. It is normal for iron to turn your stools black. Like other vitamins and minerals, very high doses of iron can be toxic.

Medical Treatments. Depending on the severity of the changes, most women we spoke with were able to find ways of coping

53

with the uncertainty and inconvenience they sometimes cause. However, do not ignore breakthrough bleeding, which may be a symptom of cancer in the reproductive organs, or heavy bleeding which could lead to anemia. If you have spotting or bleeding between periods (breakthrough bleeding), very heavy bleeding or bleeding after intercourse, you should consult a doctor.

When investigating menstrual problems, the doctor should consider the complete medical situation in order to make a proper assessment. This is done during an office visit which includes a gynecological exam and possibly other tests and procedures. These are all described in Parts 3 and 4 of this book.

Drugs and surgery are the most common treatments for flooding and/or breakthrough bleeding. The drug treatment makes use of hormones. When a woman has very heavy periods or flooding, a low dose of progesterone is prescribed for 10 days, usually beginning around day 15 of the menstrual cycle. This is the time that ovulation would usually happen and progesterone secretion would start. The progesterone allows the endometrium to develop in an orderly way; the period which follows may be heavy, but the one after that should be more manageable, with normal flow. This procedure, repeated over a few cycles, may be sufficient to stop the flooding or breakthrough bleeding, sometimes permanently. Or it may return, and hormones are tried again or surgery is considered.

Dilatation and Curettage (D&C)(see page 101) is a surgical intervention used to diagnose the reason for abnormal bleeding. The endometrial lining is scraped and the tissue which is removed is examined in a laboratory for signs of cancer or other possible causes of the bleeding. D&C also works as a temporary treatment because once the overgrowth

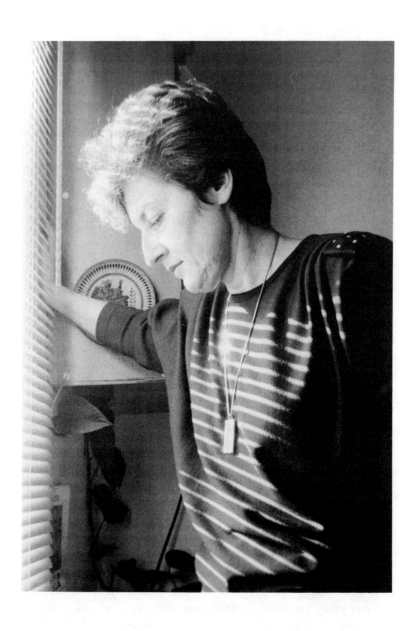

of endometrium is gone, months or even years can pass without the problem recurring. Sometimes this is long enough to get a woman past her menopause. However, some women require a few D&C's to manage the flooding before they reach menopause.

Aspiration (see page 104) is now replacing the D&C in certain centres; it is simpler and can be done in the doctor's office under local anesthetic. The risks of anesthesia and the costs of treatment are greatly reduced.

Some gynecologists are experimenting with Laser therapy to destroy overgrown endometrial tissue which is causing bleeding. This treatment is not widely available.

Hysterectomy (removal of the uterus) may be proposed as a permanent solution to the problem of pre-menopausal menstrual changes. In some situations this is the only useful solution. However, the frequency with which hysterectomy is recommended reflects of the belief that the uterus is a useless organ once childbearing is over. In fact, there is more and more evidence that this is false. The uterus plays an important role in sexuality for many women. It affects their experience of excitation and orgasm.

Hysterectomy is major surgery with both short and long-term consequences. (see Part 3 — Hysterectomy and Surgical Menopause). The decision to choose such a radical solution to a short-term problem should be considered very carefully, and should be based on solid information.

HOT FLASHES

"It starts at your toes and it just goes up. Your blood boils. You feel like you are on fire. My face gets red, red. And then you sweat. Your hair is all wet. If you are sleeping it will wake you up. You uncover and a few minutes after you get chills because you are wet and you were so hot. They last four or five minutes maybe. Maybe not that long but it seems long. I used to get them — my

goodness — I could get ten within an hour. It used to be so bad."

What Are They?

If there is a single symbol that represents menopause it is the hot flash. For many of us, menopause starts when the flashes begin and finishes when they are over. This is because they are so common and unlike anything most of us have ever experienced. Because the flushing and sweating are sometimes visible to others, hot flashes identify us as "menopausal".

Hot flashes are described as a feeling of intense heat that spreads across the upper body, neck and head. They last anywhere from 30 seconds to a few minutes and are often accompanied by a fast heart beat, sweating and flushing of the chest, face and neck.

No two women experience hot flashes in the same way. Some flashes are mild enough to be almost unrecognizable. Others are intense and unmistakable. Some women have a veritable river of sweat running down their back or chest, while others have slight dew on the bridge of their nose. Some never sweat at all. Some women have warning signs that a hot flash is about to happen — a mild tingling in the hands or feet, or throbbing in the head. Others have a general sense that a flash is coming but without any specific sign.

Hot flashes happen most often at night, and in the early morning and late evening. Those that occur during sleep are called night sweats. Women wake up kicking off their blankets and jump up to throw open the windows. Some women sweat so heavily that they have to change their night clothes and bedding before they can get back to sleep.

Frequent night sweats may cause major disruptions in your sleep cycle which can have a significant impact on your life. They can lead to exhaustion, and sometimes to anxiety or depression. Night sweats can also put stress on the relationship with a bed partner who is awakened to have sheets changed or is coping with open bedroom windows on cold winter nights!

Most women who get hot flashes have them for 1 to 5 years, starting before menopause and ending a few years after the last period. Some women have them for only a few weeks, and at the other extreme some have them for 5 to 10 years or even longer.

Who Gets Them?

"I have friends who get them severely but I don't. Still, I can't even look a sweater in the face."

It is not known exactly how many women experience hot flashes. Estimates based on studies range from 65% to 90%. Certainly the majority of us will have some experience with hot flashes. Women who have had a surgical menopause (i.e. have had their ovaries removed before going through natural menopause), are more likely to have severe and frequent hot flashes after the surgery.

Why Do They Happen?

During a hot flash the blood vessels just below the skin surface dilate or widen. This causes more blood to rush to the skin surface making it feel warm and flushed. The body responds by sweating, to cool itself down. This is the body's normal response to heat, either external — on a hot and humid day, or internal — when we have a fever. What is unusual about hot flashes is that this process is set into motion for no apparent reason. There is no fever and no hot summer day.

No one knows what signals the body that it is hot or why hot flashes happen. Although they are believed to be related in some way to the hormonal fluctuations of the peri-menopausal

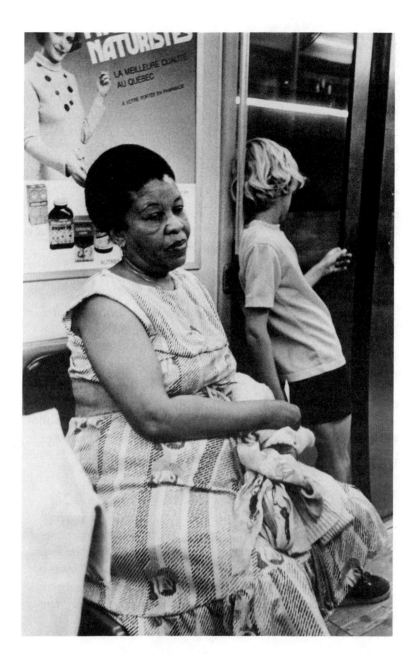

period, the exact relationship between the two is unclear. The currently accepted theory is that the hormonal imbalance in the hypothalamus caused by fluctuating FSH and estrogen levels causes the flashes. It seems logical that the hypothalamus might be involved because the body's temperature control center is located there. Estrogen levels are decreased and FSH levels increased in women who have hot flashes. A surge of LH precedes a flash.

Coping With The Changes

Reactions to hot flashes are as variable as the flashes themselves. The frequency and intensity of flashes and when they occur are key factors in determining how we cope.

"I felt miserable about the hot flashes. That was the worst part. It was much worse than the periods ending. But I didn't do anything. I just lived with it. I didn't run to the doctor."

Only 20% of North American women are so troubled by their hot flashes that they need to consult a doctor about them. Some see them as a nuisance, while others take a more philosophical approach, viewing them as symbolic of this stage in their lives.

"I took some courses in relaxation techniques. They really are wonderfully effective. I practice them when I feel a flash coming on. You sort of center your concentration on relaxing your whole body, and release the tension. And I wear cotton sleep wear and I keep a towel by the bed to rub myself down during the night. I keep away from coffee and stimulants. And liquor seems to be the worst thing."

Helping Ourselves. If you have hot flashes and find them distressing, there are many strategies you can try for dealing with them. These can be as simple as sucking on an ice cube to cool off during a hot flash or as involved as using biofeedback to will the flashes away. Some women report that regular exercise decreases the number of hot flashes; others use yoga or relaxation techniques.

Simple remedies can make a big difference. Clothes made of natural fibers are more absorbent and breathe more. They feel more comfortable during a hot flash. Wearing layers of clothes which can be peeled down to a light cotton shirt at the first sign of a hot flash may also help. Ask other women what tricks they use and which ones work best.

If you find your flashes are triggered by certain things such as alcohol, caffeine, chocolate or spicy foods, you could try reducing or eliminating them. Try sleeping with a light blanket rather than luxuriating under winter quilts.

Some women deal with their hot flashes through *acupuncture* or *acupressure*. These ancient Chinese treatments have recently become popular in North America. Acupuncture involves the insertion of tiny needles at specific points on the body. Acupressure focuses on the same points using massage or pressure rather than needles. Acupuncture should be done by qualified professionals. Acupressure is a technique that some women do for themselves or each other, but it makes sense to first learn the proper technique from an expert.

Biofeedback involves concentrating on the sensation of the hot flash and willing away the blood vessel changes and the sensation of heat that accompanies them. Biofeedback may also be useful in controlling migraines and high blood pressure.

Vitamin E, probably the best known of the natural remedies for hot flashes, has had an interesting history. A number of studies done in the 1930s and 40s showed that Vitamin E was effective in treating some of the symptoms of menopause including hot flashes. The treatment went out of style until the

1970s when a magazine survey asked readers about their use of Vitamin E. Although menopause was not specifically mentioned in the questions, 2000 women responded that Vitamin E helped relieve their hot flashes!

Vitamin E has a large group of believers and an equally large group of skeptics. Because it has been touted as a cure for so many conditions, people are suspicious when yet another use for it is proposed. Also, the profits that drug companies stand to make from widespread use of any vitamin or other drug trigger wariness in many people.

Women who try Vitamin E should do so for a few weeks to see whether it is going to work for them. Even when effective it may only help temporarily and may not eliminate the flashes completely.

Women with high blood pressure, diabetes or rheumatic heart disease should not take high doses. As with any other fat soluble vitamins (ones that dissolve in fatty tissue and are stored in the body), Vitamin E is toxic in high doses.

Ginseng is another popular natural remedy. Some people say it has a synergistic effect when taken with Vitamin E (the combined effect is greater than the individual strengths of each one). Ginseng is available in various forms at health food stores and some pharmacies.

Medical Treatments. If your hot flashes are terribly disruptive and non-prescription remedies provide little relief, you may turn to a doctor for medication. Three medications are used to treat hot flashes: estrogen (in the form of HRT), Dixarit and Bellergal.

HRT is by far the most effective treatment for hot flashes. In fact most women report that the flashes begin to disappear within hours of starting treatment, and are eventually completely eliminated in almost all cases. But HRT carries risks, and cannot be used by everyone. There is much debate over when and for how long it should be given, and the flashes sometimes return when the treatment is stopped. The use of HRT is a complex and controversial issue and is discussed fully in Part 3.

Dixarit is a prescription drug available in Canada, which is sometimes used to treat flashes but not other menopausal symptoms. A low dose of the drug Clonidine which is used to treat high blood pressure, Dixarit is believed to control hot flashes by acting directly on blood vessels. There is

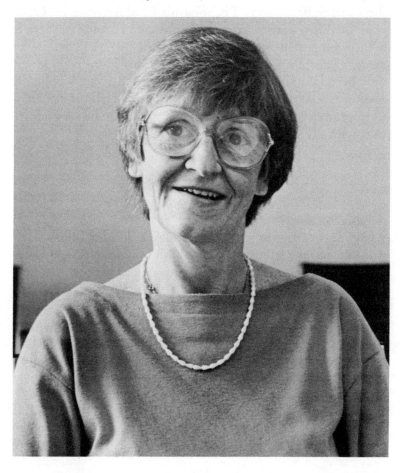

disagreement among both women who use it and doctors who prescribe it as to how well it works. Even among those who feel it works well, many find its effects are only temporary.

Dixarit causes a drying of the mucous membranes of the nose, mouth and eyes. Also, it may lower blood pressure slightly. If you already have low blood pressure you should get up slowly after lying or sitting and get out of a hot bathtub carefully so as not to feel faint.

The third drug that is used is *Bellergal*, a combination of three drugs: Belladonna, Phenobarbital and Ergotamine. Once promoted for women who could not take hormones, there is no proof that Bellergal works, and it is rarely mentioned in the newer gynecology textbooks. Bellergal should be avoided not only because of its ineffectiveness, but also because it contains phenobarbital, a tranquillizer (barbiturate). Barbiturates, used to treat anxiety, have major side effects and can be very addictive, with severe withdrawal symptoms.

VAGINAL CHANGES

What Are They?
After menopause the walls of the vagina become thinner, and produce fewer secretions. Vaginal lubrication with sexual excitement occurs more slowly. If you are accustomed to examining yourself, you may notice that your vagina is paler and the walls smoother, without the many folds typical of the reproductive years. The lips of your vulva may be thinner and flatter. As the amount of estrogen decreases, your vagina becomes less acidic making you more susceptible to vaginal infection, including yeast infections. In later years, your vagina may shorten and narrow.

You probably won't notice mild changes in the thickness and elasticity of your vaginal walls. If changes are more significant, you may have a feeling of dryness or irritation. Severe

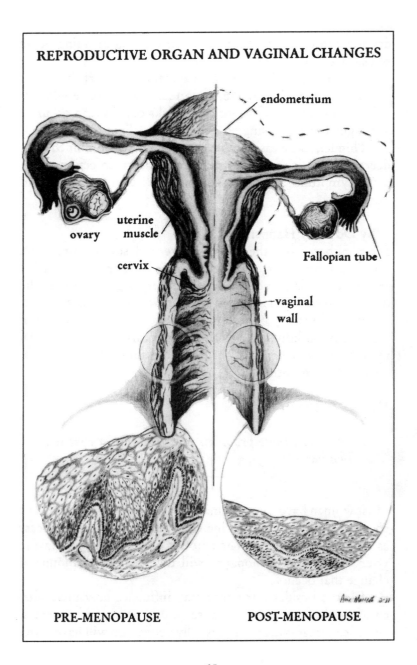

REPRODUCTIVE ORGAN AND VAGINAL CHANGES

endometrium

ovary   uterine
         muscle

cervix

Fallopian tube

vaginal
wall

PRE-MENOPAUSE   POST-MENOPAUSE

dryness can cause vaginal pain when walking or doing other physical activity.

You are most likely to feel vaginal discomfort during or just after sexual intercourse. If you have intercourse without being wet enough, abrasions (tiny nicks or cuts) can occur in the vaginal walls causing pain or spotting (light bleeding).

Thinner, more easily injured vaginal tissue combined with decreased acidity of the vagina can lead to infections. The usual symptoms are increased vaginal discharge, itching and burning.

Why Do They Happen?
From puberty on, the reproductive and sexual organs are nourished by estrogen. The decrease in estrogen levels at menopause brings about changes in these organs. Because the decrease in estrogen is a slow process, vaginal changes happen slowly, and usually become noticeable five to ten years after menopause although they can happen earlier. After surgical menopause they happen more quickly, sometimes after only six to twelve months.

Who Gets Them?

"I never had those problems of a dry vagina that some women have."

Most women have some vaginal changes after menopause. The changes progress with age since the levels of estrogen decrease as a woman gets older. The amount of estrogen you have in your blood after menopause will determine the amount of change that occurs.

Factors besides hormones may influence how much discomfort the changes will cause you. For example there is evidence that if you remain sexually active you will have fewer

66

vaginal problems than if you are celibate or only have occasional sex. Regular sexual activity, either with a partner or by masturbation, seems to increase both the amount of lubrication and the ease with which you become lubricated during sexual excitement.

Coping With The Changes

Helping Ourselves. It can be very reassuring to those of us who remain sexually active to know that having regular sex may actually reduce our risk of vaginal problems and enhance our sex lives. Although sexual activity helps keep the vagina healthy, it should not be prescribed as if it were some kind of medication. The "use it or lose it" approach is disheartening to those of us who are not comfortable with masturbation, who choose not to be sexually active or who have no available partner. We have the right to find our own sexual pace and to change that pace when we want, without being made to feel that we have created our own problems.

The positive benefits of sexual activity are not lost forever after a period of abstinence. As long as you resume intercourse gradually and carefully, you can avoid injury to your vaginal tissue; after a few weeks of regular sexual activity, lubrication and elasticity should increase.

Slower love-making is often enough to remedy the problem of vaginal pain during sex because it allows more time for natural lubrication before penetration. If you find you are not wet enough even when aroused you can try out different kinds of extra lubrication. Saliva works well for some women. Water soluble jellies such as KY Jelly are available in pharmacies without a prescription. Or you might experiment with natural oils such as almond or safflower oil. Vaseline and other petroleum-based products should not be used in the vagina because they clog the mucous membranes and are not easily washed away by the vaginal secretions.

67

FOR A FLOWERING VAGINAL FLORA

After urination and bowel movements, always wipe from front to back. Bacteria found near the rectum can cause infection if they come in contact with the vaginal opening.

- If you have sensitive skin, avoid using perfumed soaps and bath oils which can cause irritation.

- Avoid commercial feminine hygiene products which are promoted to cover up and eliminate normal vaginal odours and prevent infection. These chemicals irritate the vagina and cause infection.

- Avoid frequent douching which can wash away the normal protective bacteria in the vagina.

- Wear underwear, pantyhose and tights with a cotton crotch which allows good air flow and thus discourages bacterial growth.

- Avoid sexual intercourse if it causes pain. Use some kind of water-soluble lubrication if necessary to prevent injury to vaginal tissue.

- Plain, unsweetened yoghurt or yoghurt capsules which are available in pharmacies or natural food stores can be inserted in the vagina to help maintain or restore the natural bacterial balance. Be sure the product you use contains acidophilus or lactobacillus. Natural yoghurt can be inserted with an empty tampon inserter, vaginal cream inserter or the like. Diaphragm jelly inserters can be bought at the pharmacy without having to buy the jelly. Insert the yoghurt at bedtime. You may need to wear a pad in the morning.

We use lubricating jelly and that helps. It's not that I don't have sufficient lubrication, but the cream adds just enough extra so that I'm less tense — less worried that it might be uncomfortable, and subsequently my husband is less tense too.

Medical Treatment. If you have recurring vaginal infections, a diagnosis of the cause can be made by examining a sample of discharge under the microscope to look for yeast or bacteria. Sometimes a sample must be sent to a lab. If your doctor does not have access to a microscope find one who does; it is usually not sufficient to guess at the cause of the infection based on the colour of the discharge or other symptoms. Guessing often results in misdiagnoses, incorrect treatment and recurrences of the infection.

Treatment depends on the exact diagnosis. Local treatments such as creams and suppositories are used for yeast infections, whereas antibiotics, either in cream or pill form are used for bacterial infections. The treatment for vaginal infection is usually effective, but infections often recur if the situation which led to them continues. Unfortunately infections are not always preventable, but some basic precautions may help.

If your life is severely disrupted by vaginal symptoms and you have not been able to find relief through other means, you could consider hormone treatment. By reintroducing the hormonal stimulation to your vagina the thinning, drying and loss of elasticity can be reversed. This helps with problems of increased vaginal infections, feelings of dryness and irritation, and pain and bleeding with intercourse. Sometimes the doctor will prescribe hormones on the basis of your description of the problem and a pelvic examination. Other doctors will prepare a slide of vaginal cells (much like a Pap test), to look at under the microscope. Cells stimulated by high levels of estrogen look different from cells that aren't. This slide test is an inexpensive way of determining your menopausal status and can be helpful in making the decision whether to take hormones.

Estrogen cream used for a short time or from time to time is often adequate to bring short-term relief of vaginal symptoms. You may have to take it longer — 6 months or a year, to sufficiently reverse the vaginal changes so that the effects will be more long-lasting.

"A year and a half ago my doctor noted thinning of my vaginal walls and he gave me estrogen cream, which really works. I've had much less discomfort with intercourse. He told me to keep doing it every month for a week, but I didn't want to do that. I stopped after one month and it was quite a few months before I started getting irritation with intercourse again."

The decision to use hormones and in what form (pills, creams, etc.) is discussed in detail in Part 3 – Hormone Replacement Therapy.

OSTEOPOROSIS

"I retired in September and that January I couldn't get out of bed. It was in my back and neck. I went to England in May and had to wear a collar the whole time even to sleep. Then I went to the doctor and he sent me to a physiotherapist but it took me a long time to get supple again. Then they decided to x-ray and found me full of osteoporosis. That is why he put me on Premarin. He said it won't hurt you because you've had a hysterectomy, and we'll also give you calcium for the bones."

What Is It?
Osteoporosis is a common, but serious and debilitating disorder in which bones become porous, fragile and easily broken. Osteoporosis is a more pronounced and severe form of the bone loss which occurs in all men and women with age; unlike this universal bone loss, it is not an automatic part of aging.

Bone is made up of many different minerals, of which

calcium is the most important. Our bodies contain two types of bone: cortical bone — the long shiny bones of our arms and legs, and trabecular bone — the porous, rough bones of our torso, spine and hips. Trabecular bone in particular is affected by osteoporosis.

It is easy to think of our skeleton as something which

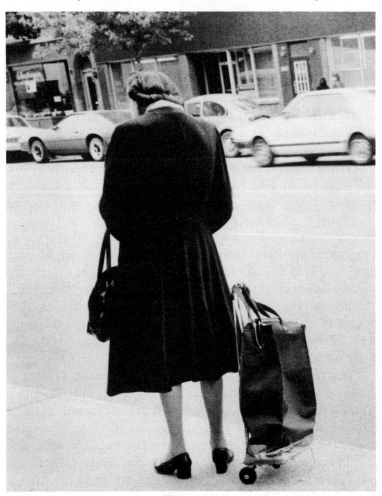

remains unchanged once we have finished growing. In fact, bone is very much "alive". In a process called remodelling, new bone is constantly formed and old bone is broken down (resorbed). Bone remodelling goes on all our lives. It is the process responsible for healing of bone that has been broken. But as we get older the ratio of bone formation to resorption shifts. When we are still growing and in our early adult years, formation happens more quickly than resorption, and our bone mass increases. Men and women reach their peak bone mass in their thirties. After that the balance between formation and resorption reverses, and bone mass begins to decrease. Osteoporotic bone does not look different from the outside unless there has been a break. Only when you cut across the bone can you see gaps in the structure. Healthy bone looks like ivory, while osteoporotic bone looks like a sponge.

There are few early warning signs of osteoporosis. We usually first find out about it when we break a bone. A common complication is compression fractures of the spine which begin to occur around age 50 or 60. These fractures happen during normal activity without a fall or other trauma. They cause persistent lower back pain and loss of height; over time they lead to a distinctive hump in the back, sometimes called a dowager's hump. Eventually the spine bends forward coming to rest on the hips, and can compress the internal organs of the abdomen (see the diagram on page 74). With severe osteoporosis, you can lose as much as eight inches of body height.

Wrist fractures are also common and begin to occur around the same age as compression fractures. They can result from a fall or a simple banging of your wrist against something. The hip is another common site of fractures. Broken hips were once thought to occur as a result of a fall, but now we know that in some cases the hip breaks spontaneously, causing the fall. Hip fractures often require surgery, which in the elderly has a high (10 – 20%) mortality rate.

Who Gets It?

"I take OSCAL, 500 mg daily. My mother broke her hip, quite by accident. She was taking a fitness class, tripped and broke her hip. We didn't know that she had osteoporosis but she must have."

Although certain diseases and prolonged immobility can lead to osteoporosis, it is primarily a condition of post-menopausal women. Approximately 25% of post-menopausal North American women develop osteoporosis.

We still have much to learn about what differentiates those 25% from the 75% who do not get it. Of the risk factors that have been identified, some are outside our control. For example some of us are genetically more susceptible. Other risk factors have more to do with lifestyle choices over which we do have control, such as smoking, alcohol, caffeine and exercise. How these factors interact with each other is not clear. Nor is their relative importance in the development of osteoporosis. Those of us with multiple risk factors should be especially concerned about prevention. What are the risk factors?

Genetic Factors. If your mother or sister has osteoporosis you have an increased risk of developing it. Caucasian women, especially those who are fair-skinned, small-boned and from a northern European ancestry are also at greater risk. Black women have greater bone mass than white women and rarely develop osteoporosis.

Nutritional Factors. Our bodies use calcium for bone formation but calcium has other functions as well. When calcium levels in the blood are not high enough to carry out these functions, the body takes it from bone. Our bodies do not make calcium, so we must get it from the food we eat. A diet

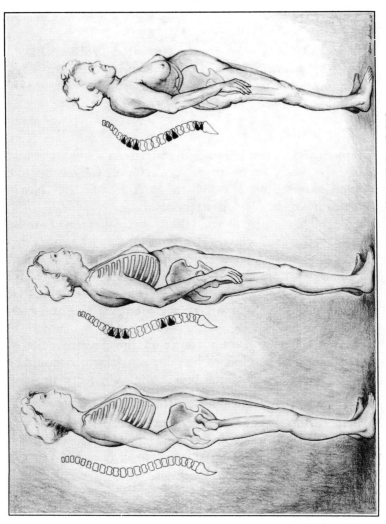

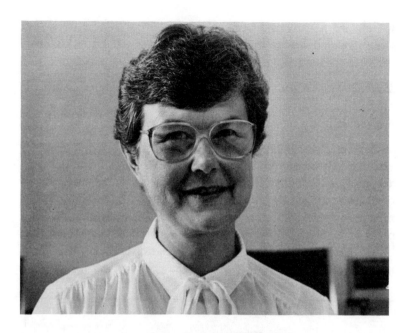

low in calcium increases the risk for osteoporosis.

Vitamin D is essential for the absorption of calcium. Sunshine is the best source of this vitamin. With fifteen minutes of exposure, our bodies produce enough vitamin D for a day. Most commercial dairies add vitamin D to their milk, so there is little risk of vitamin D deficiency in our culture. Theoretically, if you live through northern winters where the sun is weak and your skin is covered most of the time, and you do not drink vitaminized milk, you might not get enough of this vitamin. In reality though, this problem is rare.

Protein increases the excretion of calcium from the body in the urine. Phosphates contained in red meat decrease calcium absorption from the intestines. A diet very high in animal protein has been shown to contribute to bone loss in animals, and research is underway to see if it does the same in people.

Constant dieting is also a risk factor for osteoporosis. When dieting we tend to avoid "fattening" dairy products

75

which are among the best calcium sources. The low body weight which we are trying to achieve is in itself a risk factor for osteoporosis.

Low Body Weight. Because one of the primary sources of estrogen after menopause is fatty tissue (see page 33), women with little body fat have lower levels of estrogen.

Sedentary Lifestyle. At all ages exercise increases bone mass. If you are physically active you will have greater bone density and muscle mass than if you remain sedentary. Exercise affects bone by straining the muscles which support the skeleton. The muscles in turn put stress on the bones. Like a see-saw, muscle pulls on bone and bone resists. This resistance strengthens the bone. Without this kind of regular exercise, osteoporosis is more likely to develop.

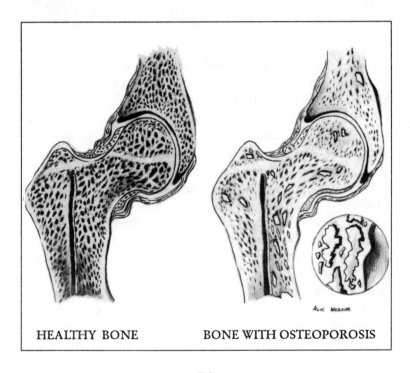

HEALTHY BONE   BONE WITH OSTEOPOROSIS

RISK FACTORS FOR OSTEOPOROSIS

High Risk	High Risk But Preventable
family history	diet consistently low in calcium
age	sedentary lifestyle
Caucasian	smoking
small bones	heavy drinking
fair skin	high caffeine intake
early menopause (natural	high protein diet
or surgical)	low body weight
certain diseases (see text)	constant dieting
regular use of steroids	diet low in vitamin D

Early Menopause. Menopause speeds up the rate of bone loss for all women, with the greatest amount of loss happening in the first few years after menopause. Those whose menopause occurs early (before the late 40s), either naturally or due to surgery, are at greater risk because they will have more years post-menopause without the protective effect of estrogen on their bones.

Smoking. Smoking affects osteoporosis, but the exact relationship is not clearly understood. It probably has a direct effect on the body's use or absorption of calcium. Smoking also brings on an earlier natural menopause.

Alcohol and Caffeine. In some studies, heavy intake of both of these drugs has been associated with decreased bone mass.

General Health Factors. Certain diseases predispose a woman to osteoporosis including inflammatory bowel disease, some thyroid disease and chronic liver and kidney disease. If you regularly use steroid medications such as cortisone, you are also at greater risk.

Why Does It Happen?

"I have an illness which makes me more susceptible to osteoporosis, so I am concerned about it. But I haven't considered Premarin for prevention because I'm scared of it. I weigh osteoporosis against some form of cancer, stroke, heart disease. Also, because I'm already on so much medication it makes the idea of Premarin more difficult to deal with."

High rates of osteoporosis in post-menopausal women are linked to their decreased estrogen levels. Estrogen has a protective effect on bones. It blocks another hormone (parathyroid hormone) from stimulating bone resorption. With less estrogen, bone-mass loss accelerates for 5 to 10 years after menopause. Together with the normal decrease in bone mass which happens with aging, this puts about one quarter of us at risk of developing fractures after menopause.

Coping With The Changes

Osteoporosis often goes unnoticed until you begin to have back pain or fall and break a bone. Because there are no early warning signs and no simple tests, it is very important for all of us to evaluate our chances of developing osteoporosis.

Ordinary X-rays do not detect osteoporosis until it is very advanced. Some doctors have access to specialized machines that measure bone density to diagnose osteoporosis and evaluate the effectiveness of therapy. However, the machines are expensive and not widely available. More important, their results do not really change the approach to the problem.

Two critical issues surround osteoporosis. The first is whether it can be prevented, and if so, how. Will a prevention program, for example, be useful for a woman at high risk of developing osteoporosis, or only for those at low risk? The second question is whether it is possible to treat osteoporosis, i.e. to restore lost bone. These questions are being studied extensively. At this point there is more controversy than clear-cut answers.

If a preventive program is started early enough, osteoporosis may be preventable. We can even prevent further bone loss after we have already had fractures due to osteoporosis. However, no treatment has been proven to restore lost bone. What we as individuals choose to do in the face of osteoporosis will be based on our own risk factors, our general health, and our personal values and lifestyle.

"I walk briskly every day and I ride a bike everywhere I can. We never take the car if we can help it. I've made an effort to drink more milk and eat more cheese. With all the osteoporosis information virtually flooding the popular press, I guess I am a bit concerned."

Helping Ourselves. A decision to try to prevent osteoporosis is in essence a decision to change some or all of our preventable risk factors (see chart, page 77). The two most important preventive measures we can take are in the areas of diet and exercise.

Diet. Since our bodies do not manufacture calcium, we depend on a well-balanced diet to meet our needs. Yet many of us decrease our intake of dairy products as we get older. The amount of calcium available in the blood stream for bone remodelling is reduced even more as our bodies age because our intestines absorb less calcium.

We do not yet know for certain whether adding large amounts of calcium to our diet during and after menopause will actually lead to that calcium being deposited in our bones. How much calcium we really need each day remains controversial. There is agreement though that adequate calcium intake by young women is critical for strong bones later in life, and that by the time we reach mid-life few of us are getting enough calcium. It is currently recommended that pre-menopausal women take 800 mg and post-menopausal women 1200 – 1500 mg daily. Women taking hormones probably only need 1000 mg daily, since calcium is more effective when combined with hormone replacement therapy.

In order not to trade one health risk for another, try to get your calcium from low fat dairy products. Low fat yoghurt and cheese, as well as 2% or skim milk, are all excellent sources of calcium.

If you are unable to maintain a diet rich enough in calcium you may decide to take calcium supplements. There are many different kinds available, and the costs and contents vary. The form of calcium varies from supplement to supplement, and some contain other vitamins as well, including vitamin D. Calcium carbonate provides the most usable calcium per pill. Women with an intolerance to lactose, the principle sugar found in milk and some other dairy products, should avoid calcium lactate. Calcium chloride causes more side effects including gas, bloating and cramping, but any of the calciums can have this effect. Experiment with different brands until you find one that suits you. If you are already susceptible to developing kidney stones you should not take high doses of

---

Aggressive advertising campaigns promoting calcium supplements have followed close on the heels of medical interest in the prevention of osteoporosis. Once again the drug companies are cashing in on menopause, moulding public knowledge and opinion in the process. Their advertisements in medical journals and women's magazines, on TV and radio, all proclaim calcium as a sure method of preventing osteoporosis. But the research results are inconclusive. Although we may be helping ourselves by increasing our calcium intake, we definitely are helping the drug companies make a profit. The possibility remains that we may be spending large sums of money for little or no effect.

FOODS THAT ARE HIGH IN CALCIUM

	AMOUNT	CALCIUM*
Yoghurt	250 ml (1 cup)	352 mg
Cheddar cheese	45 g (1.5 oz)	324 mg
Milk (skim)	250 ml (1 cup)	317 mg
Milk (2%)	250 ml (1 cup)	315 mg
Milk (whole)	250 ml (1 cup)	306 mg
Tahini	60 ml (4 tbsp)	270 mg
Ice Cream	250 ml (1 cup)	184 mg
Almonds	125 ml (1/2 cup)	175 mg
Cottage Cheese (2%)	250 ml (1 cup)	161 mg
Broccoli	1 stalk	158 mg
Blackstrap Molasses	15 ml (1 tbsp)	137 mg
Canned Salmon (& bones)	125 ml (1/2 cup)	125 mg

* Figures taken from *Health and Welfare Canada*, Nutrient Value of Some Common Foods

calcium. Remember, no amount of calcium will maintain the bone mass of a sedentary person.

In addition to increasing your calcium intake, you can also avoid doing things which decrease calcium absorption or increase its excretion from the body. This includes stopping smoking, cutting down on alcohol and caffeine, and not getting too many of your daily calories from protein.

If you are not getting vitamin D in your milk, and you are not often out in the sun, you might consider a supplement (400 I.U.). Vitamin D supplements should be used with caution because high doses can actually cause loss of bone mass. Over 4000 I.U. can be toxic.

Menopause is a good time to reconsider the virtues of being skinny. An obsession with being slim diminishes the chance of maintaining healthy bone because it further reduces your levels of estrogen and its protective effect on your bones. We are not promoting obesity which carries other health risks. The goal is a comfortable weight for our height, frame and body type.

Insurance companies recently revised their ideal weight scales, realizing that contrary to popular belief, you can be too thin. Many of us are pleasantly surprised to find out that we are indeed a good healthy weight after years of thinking we had a few pounds to lose.

Exercise. There is no question that a sedentary lifestyle increases the risk of osteoporosis. Exercise increases bone density. It

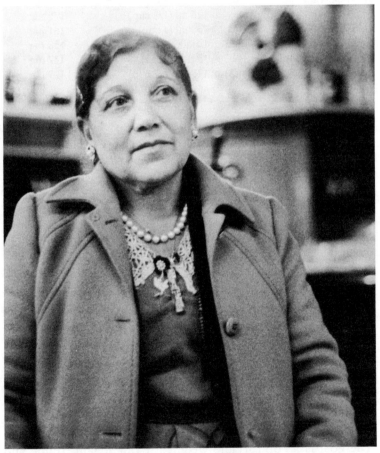

may also help to protect bone mass by increasing the production of estrogen, which is important to bone maintenance. Exercise makes us more agile and therefore less prone to falling. Exercise combats osteoporosis only if it is weight-bearing exercise. That means exercise in which you carry your own weight and/or extra weight, for example walking, dancing, skiing and biking. Exercise in which you are weightless, for example swimming, does not have the same effect on bone mass, but has other benefits.

Medical Treatments

Hormone Replacement Therapy. HRT, or more specifically the estrogen part of the therapy, is used sometimes to prevent osteoporosis. It stabilizes bone loss and maintains the bones at a level of density that will prevent fractures. Whether it actually rebuilds lost bone is a hotly debated question. There is an increasing tendency to use long-term hormone therapy for women at high risk. HRT is most often recommended to women who have a very early menopause or a strong family history of osteoporosis. Some doctors recommend that all women take it regardless of their relative risk. We believe that this decision should be considered carefully, weighing your personal risk factors against the risks of the treatment (see page 134 for risks of HRT).

There is not yet agreement as to the best type of estrogen, the exact regimen or even the best form in which to take hormones to prevent osteoporosis. The earlier in the post-menopausal period you start the treatment the better, since bone loss begins quickly. The hormones are continued for an extended period — possibly for the rest of your life since some studies show an accelerated bone loss in women who stop taking the hormones. The critical question to which we do not yet have the answer is whether this accelerated loss is sufficient to undo the good of several years of hormone use. Knowing this would be the key to deciding how long medication is necessary.

Fluoride. Fluoride is used experimentally in the treatment of osteoporosis. It increases the formation of new bone. However the quality of the new bone is questionable and whether it is resistant to fractures is not yet clear. Some recent studies suggest that fluoride may strengthen trabecular bone, but weaken cortical bone. This means you would be less likely to break your hip, but more likely to break a leg.

Calcitonin. Calcitonin is a hormone produced by the thyroid gland which contributes to bone formation. Levels of calcitonin gradually decrease with age. Calcitonin injections have been tried on an experimental basis to treat osteoporosis. It appears that women develop resistance to the drug within twelve to eighteen months, and at that point the treatment stops being effective.

BEYOND THE "BIG FOUR": OTHER CHANGES

"If I had to describe it to my daughters, it's like having premenstrual tension all the time."

What Are They?
Menstrual cycle changes, hot flashes, vaginal changes and osteoporosis are "the big four" of menopause. Although not all women experience them, it is widely accepted that they are caused by hormonal changes related to menopause. Yet many of us experience other physical and emotional changes that we associate with menopause. The women we spoke with talked about migraines and other headaches, aching joints, insomnia, fatigue, anxiety, irritability, depression and bloating. Symptom checklists devised by researchers include still more poten-

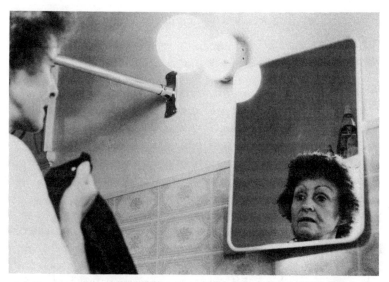

tial "symptoms" of menopause. Depression and anxiety are mentioned most frequently.

"I have lots of headaches, an increase over 5 years ago. The kind that comes and goes. It can be there for 5 minutes and disappear, and then come back half an hour later."

Depression is a mood of sadness and emotional upset. It varies from the mild and transient "blues" most of us experience at one time or another to severe incapacitating depression, where we lose all hope and cannot carry on with our lives. We may even consider or attempt suicide. Some depressions seem to occur for no apparent reason; some are caused by unexplained biochemical changes in the brain; and others happen in response to specific events or losses. People who have been depressed before are more vulnerable to another depression.

85

In our society, depression is diagnosed more commonly in women than in men.

"I would say the depression was most intense a year or so before my period stopped and a year or two after. It wasn't a deep depression. It was almost as if you can't get up the energy to have anything matter. And that causes anxiety because when you are in a job where you have to work with people and you have to relate, it's a problem."

How can you tell if you or someone you know is depressed? People who are depressed have at least a few of the following signs: they look sad or tired; lose interest in their work and other activities; have difficulty concentrating; feel bad about themselves; lose their appetite or overeat; lose interest in sex; cry a lot; have insomnia, or wake up very early in the morning and can't get back to sleep, or sleep all day.

"There just seems to be an underlying anxiety. You can't pinpoint the reason. It may not be menopausal at all. I just say it's a new feeling."

Anxiety is a feeling of fear or tension which usually happens in response to a stressful or frightening situation. People show their anxiety in different ways. Some of us become irritable. Others develop a rapid heart beat (palpitations), have trembling hands, diarrhea, nausea and vomiting, or insomnia. A certain amount of stress is part of everyday life and is beneficial, helping us to perform better in difficult or challenging situations. However, severe anxiety has the opposite effect, interfering with our ability to function and making us feel very uncomfortable.

Who Gets Them?

"I get a little blue I suppose, but no depression."

It is difficult to get a sense of how many women experience these symptoms. In part this is due to research problems. Researchers cannot even agree on what symptoms to look at, let alone whether they are related to menopause.

Certainly the list is long enough and the variety of changes broad enough that most of us are likely to experience at least one of them during our peri-menopausal years.

The prevailing stereotype of menopausal women as depressed, crazy and self-absorbed has influenced our own expectations of what menopause will be like for us. Many of the pre-menopausal women we spoke to described depression or "going crazy" as their biggest fear about menopause, yet research shows that we are no more likely to be depressed at mid-life than at other times in our lives. In other words, depression is not an inevitable part of menopause. In fact, women in their 20s, particularly those at home with young children, have the highest rate of depression. For years a psychiatric diagnosis of "involutional melancholia" linked some depressions in mid-life women to menopause. No scientific evidence exists to support this link, and the label has been eliminated from the official handbook of psychiatric diagnoses.

Why Do They Happen?

"I get bouts of depression, but which I do not link with menopause personally. I link it much more with aging

and being more aware of vulnerability, and being more aware of loneliness also."

There is a tendency to assume that everything we experience between the ages of 40 to 60 is directly attributable to menopause. This leads us to suffer needlessly from problems that might have solutions if we would just look beyond our hormones. On the other hand, an opposite tendency to assume that nothing is related to menopause except the "big four" can be equally harmful. This approach labels as psychosomatic those physical or emotional changes for which no connection to hormones has yet been found.

We do not have an answer so far to the question "why". The possibility of a hormone connection does exist, for some but not all changes. For example, headaches and hormones may be linked. Some women who regularly get migraine headaches stop getting them when they are pregnant. Other women get migraines premenstrually. Evidence as to whether HRT improves headaches is conflicting. Perhaps a hormone other than estrogen is connected with migraines.

There is some evidence that less dream sleep (REM sleep) occurs during the peri-menopausal period. This type of sleep is essential to our feeling of well-being and rest in the morning. Some people connect these changing sleep patterns to hot flashes at night (see page 57) Others have looked at the relationship between estrogen and the levels of tryptophan, a sleep-inducing chemical in the brain.

"I would often wake up at 4:00 in the morning and I would think — oh god, I have to get up soon and I can't get back to sleep. I used to get up at 6:15 and feel dragged out."

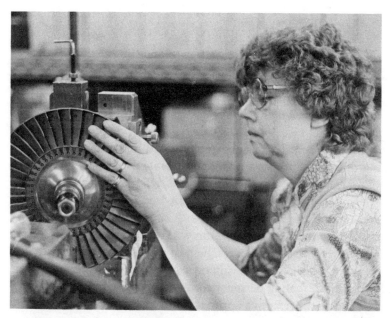

You might experience depression or anxiety at mid-life for a number of reasons. The hormonal fluctuations of menopause may be responsible. A direct hormonal connection is suggested by the fact that many women notice more marked premenstrual mood swings in the pre-menopausal years. LH may play a role in depression; depressed women have been found to have lower LH levels.

Menopause may be just one of a complex series of interrelated factors contributing to these emotional states. For example hormonal changes may decrease some women's tolerance to stressful situations in the same way that being run down decreases our resistance to catching a cold. So some of us who are used to coping with most situations find ourselves coping less effectively at mid-life. Another possible link to menopause may be night sweats which disrupt sleep and lead to symptoms of sleep deprivation (see page 56). Or, there may be absolutely no link to menopause at all. As with many other aspects of menopause, all of the evidence is not yet in.

Coping With The Changes

Helping Ourselves. Before assuming that a particular change you are experiencing is due to menopause, investigate other possible causes. In many cases the source of the problem cannot be identified. More important, it may not matter. Dealing directly with the symptom, finding a solution where possible, learning to live with it if need be, might be more useful.

When you feel depressed you can simply wait and see, while trying at the same time to be particularly nice to yourself. In some cases the situation will resolve itself in a few days or weeks. You can enlist the help of a friend or family member to listen and help you evaluate what is going on. However, if you are not feeling better within a short time, it may be better to adopt a more active approach and consult a professional.

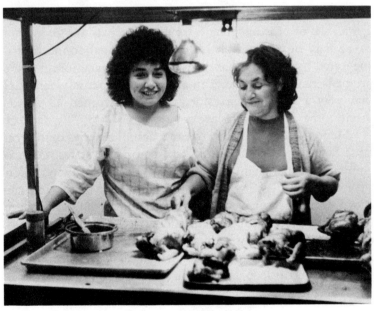

MOOD ALTERING DRUGS

ANTIDEPRESSANTS

Common names:	Elavil, Tofranil, Sinequan, Surmontil
Uses:	depression
How to take:	Start with low dose and increase weekly until it begins to work well or until it causes side effects; must be taken regularly to be effective; effects seen only after a few weeks; when feeling better, stop medication gradually.
Side effects:	Dry mouth, constipation, drowsiness, dizziness.
Addictive:	No.

ANTI-ANXIETY DRUGS (Tranquilizers) Valium-like drugs

Common names:	Valium, Librium, Dalmane, Serax, Ativan
Uses:	Anxiety, insomnia, seizures, pre-surgery sedation.
How to take:	Effective with first dose, no need to increase dose; unlike antidepressants, need not be taken regularly, but only when needed.
Side effects:	Drowsiness, listlessness, sometimes increased anxiety.
Addictive:	Yes. Long-term use can cause severe psychological and physical effects; not proven effective for over four months' use.

BARBITURATES

Common names:	Seconal, Nembutal, Amytal, Phenobarbital
Uses:	Anxiety, insomnia, seizures, pre-surgery sedation.
Side effects:	Depressed breathing, drowsiness, sometimes increased anxiety; very dangerous if taken with alcohol.
Addictive:	Yes. Withdrawal causes very severe symptoms including convulsions; easy to overdose accidentally.

Medical Treatment. Because the relationship between estrogen and many emotional changes is quite tenuous, hormone replacement therapy should be a last resort, if it is tried at all. Treatment with hormones does not usually eliminate these symptoms. When it does, the success is often considered to be due to the elimination of bothersome hot flashes.

Both anxiety and depression can be treated with prescription drugs. As a short term solution, especially in conjunction with psychotherapy, they can be very useful. But these drugs do have side effects (see page 91). Many can be addictive; when you stop taking them after a long time the withdrawal symptoms can be severe. Sometimes they have the opposite effect to that intended, making you feel even more anxious. If you notice side effects or if you feel strange while taking these medications, report the side effects to the doctor.

Mood-altering drugs are prescribed very frequently for women, much more than for men. Women working at home

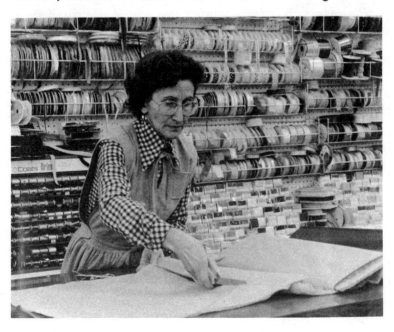

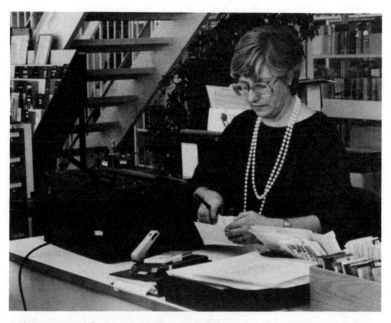

take more of these drugs than do those in the paid labour force. Elderly women are more likely to take them than younger women. And menopausal women who are anxious are sometimes given hormones with tranquilizers added to them. These drugs are frequently used to ease the pain of larger social and economic problems while avoiding the difficult and complex underlying issues. Many kinds of trained specialists are available to help you take stock of your situation and understand the reasons you are feeling the way you are. Psychologists and psychiatrists as well as some social workers, nurses, family doctors and lay therapists offer counselling services. Often these people have a specific philosophy underlying their approach. It is helpful to know something about the therapist's philosophy to assure that you will be working through your problem in a supportive and non-judgmental atmosphere, with a person who has an approach compatible with your own. Unfortunately, when we are depressed, we often do not have the energy required to shop around for the most appropriate therapist. Community groups, women's referral centres or like-minded friends may be able to provide a reference.

GENERAL BODY CHANGES

"I don't get hot flashes anymore, but I feel that my body temperature has changed. I was always too cold, I'm not anymore. Now I dress much more lightly, and prefer cotton to wool. It's not because of hot flashes, I just feel different"

The hormonal changes of menopause affect many parts of the body because both estrogen and progesterone act on so many different organs. Besides those changes commonly associated with menopause, other hormone-linked changes can occur, often not until many years after menopause. This makes it difficult to differentiate the effects of menopause from those of aging.

"I have noticed changes. My body feels different, looks different. I've much more of an appetite."

"I require less sleep, and I don't feel tired. I can stay up later at night and still wake up with lots of energy."

Ovaries and Uterus
Two kinds of change take place in the ovaries and uterus after menopause. The first change, which occurs in both the ovaries and uterus, is that they become smaller. This is triggered by the decrease in estrogen and continues over the years as part of the

normal aging process. You will not be aware of these changes yourself, but they are noticeable during a pelvic examination.

Second, some problems associated with estrogen disappear. One example is endometriosis, a condition in which endometrial tissue attaches to pelvic organs and bleeds cyclically with each month's menstrual period. Endometriosis causes severe and often debilitating menstrual pain and is a common reason for hysterectomy. The pain of endometriosis disappears with the last menstrual period.

Fibroids are non-cancerous tumors in the muscle of the uterus. They are very common and grow under the stimulation of estrogen. Small ones often go unnoticed, but if they are large, they can cause pain and very heavy periods, and can put pressure on surrounding organs. Fibroids shrink and often disappear spontaneously as estrogen levels drop after menopause.

Breasts

Breasts are made up of glands (which produce milk during breastfeeding) and fatty tissue. The glands are stimulated by both estrogen and progesterone. After menopause, when the hormonal stimulation decreases, the amount of glandular tissue decreases.

You will notice that your breasts don't feel as lumpy, due to the decrease in glandular tissue. Breast self-examination is much easier to do, as there are no longer unidentified lumps and bumps to cause anxiety. Fibrocystic Breast condition (non-cancerous breast lumps that change with the menstrual cycle) diminishes after menopause for the same reason. See Part 4 – Well Woman Care, for a discussion of breast care for mid-life women.

Urinary Tract

Like the vaginal walls, the tissue that lines the urethra (the tube which empties urine from the bladder) is stimulated by estrogen. After menopause, that tissue becomes thinner and is more easily injured, increasing the risk of developing urinary tract infections (cystitis).

The usual symptoms of infection are a feeling of having to pee often, a sense of urgency (once you need to go you wonder if you are going to make it) and burning and pain while peeing or just after. Even though the urge is very strong, there is actually very little urine.

Urinary tract infections are diagnosed by examining a sterile urine sample for the presence of bacteria and pus cells. Once an infection is diagnosed, you will be treated with antibiotics in pill form. The treatment can be given in different

---

PREVENTING URINARY TRACT INFECTIONS

After urination and bowel movements always wipe from front to back. Bacteria found near your rectum can cause infection if they come in contact with the urethral opening.

Drink lots of fluids, especially water, to help flush the urinary tract and keep it free of bacteria.

Urinate regularly. A bladder that is stretched full of urine becomes infected more easily.

Alcohol and caffeine are bladder irritants. If you get recurrent infections, try cutting down on them.

Acidic urine helps to prevent the growth of bacteria. Cranberry juice makes your urine acidic and is often recommended for preventing infections (although some people say you need to drink large volumes for it to be effective). Vitamin C, about 1000 mg. per day, also acidifies the urine.

If you are very prone to infection, positions in intercourse which put pressure on your urethra and manual or oral stimulation in the area of the urethral opening may increase the risk of infection. Urinating before and after intercourse may help. If the infections are clearly related to sexual activity, and if avoiding irritation to the urethra doesn't help, you may consider taking a single preventive dose of antibiotics either before or after having sex.

---

ways: one very large dose, several large doses or smaller doses for 7 to 10 days. You should have another sample of urine tested one week after the treatment to make sure it has worked. Otherwise the bacteria could move up to your kidneys and cause more serious illness.

If you have a lot of pain from a bladder infection you can take a pain-killing drug called pyridium for the first few days until the antibiotics begin to work. You still need to take the antibiotics because pyridium does not cure the infection. Some preparations of antibiotics also contain pyridium. This drug turns your urine bright orange or red.

One possible side effect of antibiotics is a vaginal yeast infection. Antibiotics are non-specific; they kill off not only the "bad" bacteria which cause infection, but also the "good" bacteria in the vagina which normally keep yeast under control. If you are already at risk for infections due to vaginal changes, you may want to try some of the preventive measures described on page 68. Yoghurt inserted into your vagina every night while taking the antibiotic may be especially helpful because acidophilus, the bacteria in yoghurt culture, is the

---

BURNING MOUTH SYNDROME

Burning mouth syndrome is a condition reported to dentists more than to doctors. Its symptoms include a severe burning sensation in parts of the mouth, a metallic or bitter taste and a dry mouth. The burning pain generally begins in the morning and reaches a peak in the early evening.

The cause of burning mouth syndrome is not known. A connection to menopause has been suggested for several reasons: most people who suffer from this condition are post-menopausal women (but pre-menopausal women and men get it too); often the symptoms begin around the time of menopause; and women with burning mouth syndrome tend to have severe menopausal symptoms as well.

Whatever the connection to menopause, if any, HRT does not solve the problem.

---

same bacteria which is present in the vagina and which protects it from yeast infections.

You may develop urinary tract irritation without actually having an infection. Severe cases which are due to thinning of the urethral tissue are sometimes treated with hormones.

"I know I'm not 20. I'm very aware of it. Just the fact that I'm single makes me very aware of the fact. My body is not like a 20 or 30 year old. It doesn't bother me that much for myself, but I think how others perceive me. I think I should be worthwhile. It doesn't matter if my stomach is flabby and yet I think that others are judging me that way. I suddenly become frightened that I could be discarded for a firmer person."

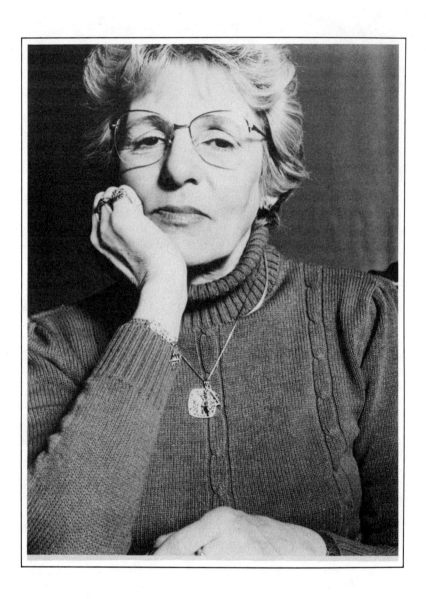

PART THREE

MEDICAL INTERVENTIONS

A lthough menopause is not a medical condition, mid-life women are subjected to an ever increasing barrage of medical procedures. It is often difficult to know whose interests are being served — the women, the doctors or the manufacturers of medical technology. This section describes briefly some of the tests used for diagnosing certain health problems in mid-life women. Two common but controversial interventions, hysterectomy and hormone replacement therapy, are discussed in greater detail.

DIAGNOSTIC TESTS

Dilatation and Curettage
A D&C is used to determine the reason for midcycle bleeding. This procedure often solves problems of heavy or irregular menstruation, at least for a short time.

A D&C is done in a hospital under general anaesthetic, while the woman is on the operating table with her legs supported in stirrups. A metal speculum is placed in the vagina;

101

DILATATION AND CURETTAGE (D & C)

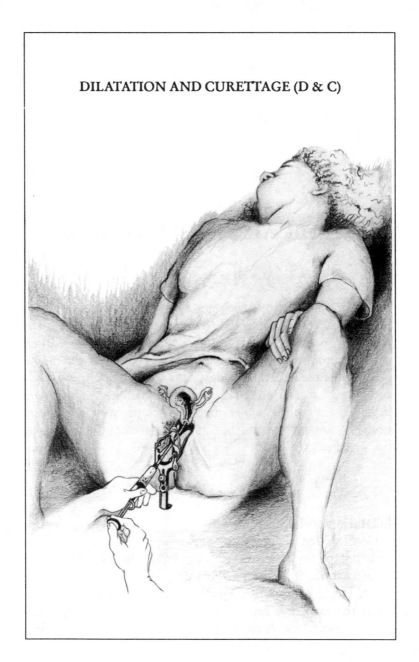

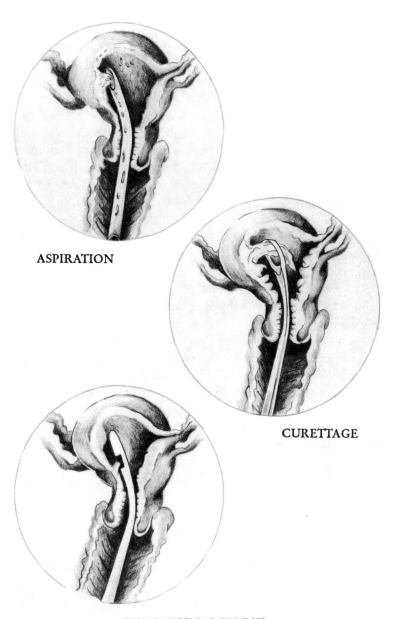

ASPIRATION

CURETTAGE

ENDOMETRIAL BIOPSY

103

the cervix is opened approximately one centimetre by inserting a series of rods (dilators) through it. A curette, which is a sharp spoon-like instrument, is inserted through the cervical opening into the uterus. The doctor uses the curette to scrape the inner walls of the uterus, removing most of the endometrial lining. This tissue is analyzed in a laboratory.

A D&C takes about 20 minutes. Cramping and bleeding are common for a few days afterward. Although considered a minor surgical procedure, a D&C does carry some risks. These include infection, perforation of the uterus, reactions to the anesthetic and accidental removal of too much endometrial lining.

Aspiration
Aspiration of the endometrial lining is rapidly replacing the D&C in testing for endometrial cancer, because it can be done in the doctor's office using local anaesthetic, and only lasts a few minutes.

A woman lies in the same position as for a routine gynecological exam. The doctor inserts a speculum and injects a local anaesthetic into the cervix. This stops the discomfort caused by the instruments themselves, but does not prevent the uterine cramps which can be mild to severe. A tube is inserted through the cervix into the uterus, usually without prior dilatation. Gentle suction is applied to remove most of the endometrial lining, which is examined later for signs of cancer. As with the D&C, cramps and bleeding are common for a few days after the procedure.

Endometrial Biopsy
This procedure, a screening test for endometrial hyperplasia (overgrowth) and endometrial cancer, is used when women have no symptoms of disease but are at risk because of the hormones they take or diseases they have. It is done under

local anaesthetic in a doctor's office and takes about 5 minutes.

A thin sharp instrument is inserted through the cervical canal and tiny bits of the uterine lining are removed to be examined under a microscope. Many women are unprepared for the sharp cramps which occur during and after the test. Most women describe it as worse than an IUD insertion, but the amount of pain is related to a number of different factors including whether the woman has ever given birth and how tense she is. There may be some spotting after the biopsy.

Pap Test

A Pap test or cytology is a screening test for cancer of the cervix. Women under 35 are counselled to have it done once a year, and less frequently with age if prior tests have been normal. Although it sometimes identifies abnormal endometrial cells which happen to be present in the cervical canal, it is not a test for endometrial cancer.

A Pap test should not be painful. A flat stick is gently rotated around the surface of the cervix; a cotton swab is similarly rotated in the cervical canal. The removed cells are spread on a small glass slide, sprayed with a fixative solution and sent to a laboratory to be examined under a microscope for signs of cellular changes or for cancer.

Colposcopy

This examination, useful for women whose Pap test is abnormal, is similar to an ordinary gynecological one except that the gynecologist looks at the cervix through a magnifying instrument (colposcope). A vinegar-like solution is applied to the cervix to make the differences between normal and abnormal cells more obvious.

If abnormal cells are seen, they can be treated immediately either with cryotherapy (freezing with liquid nitrogen) or with a laser beam. Or, a small bit of tissue can be removed (biopsied) for further evaluation before treatment.

Ultrasound

Ultrasound (echography) is a test which uses high-frequency sound waves. Similar to a ship's sonar system, ultrasound passes sound waves through the body which bounce off internal organs and produce a picture of those organs on a screen. Pelvic ultrasound is used during pregnancy, and to identify such conditions as fibroids, ovarian cysts and ovarian cancer. Because no radiation is used, ultrasound is considered a safe procedure, and there are no known harmful complications.

You need to have a full bladder during the ultrasound to facilitate the movement of the sound waves. Most women say this is the only uncomfortable part of the procedure. Lubricating jelly is applied to your lower abdomen and the transducer (the bar which emits the sound waves) is slid across your abdomen by the technician who simultaneously watches the image on the screen. Recently a new technique has been developed in which the transducer is inserted into the vagina rather than placed on the abdomen. The advantage of this newer method is that it gives more accurate images and that it does not require a full bladder.

Hysteroscopy

This examination is done by a gynecologist with special training. A telescope-like instrument is passed through the cervix into the uterus, allowing the doctor to see inside the uterus to make a diagnosis. When a larger tube is used, instruments for treatment can be passed through it. As the technology is improved, doctors are finding more uses for hysteroscopy.

Mammography

This is a breast X-ray which identifies changes in breast tissue, differentiating between types of breast disease and detecting cancerous lumps before they can be felt with the fingers.

In mammography, each breast is squeezed in turn between two flat surfaces, one of which contains the X-ray film. This is done twice for each breast, once holding the breast horizontally and once vertically, and can be uncomfortable or even painful if your breasts are tender.

Thermography
This test provides a photographic image of hot and cold spots on the surface of the breast. Because breast cancer generates higher temperature than normal tissue, it shows up as a "hot spot" on the photograph. For thermography, you will first need to sit in front of a fan with your arms raised and your breasts exposed for about five minutes to cool down your skin. The doctor or technician may examine your breasts using a light to locate clusters of veins in your breasts which could show up as false hot spots.

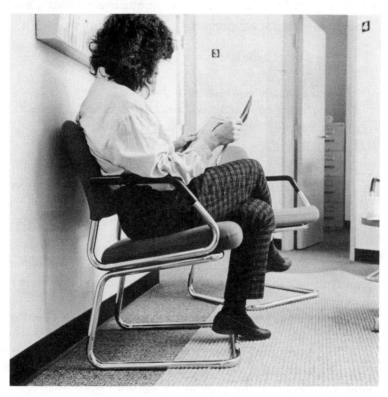

Thermography is advantageous because it does not use radiation, yet is less reliable than mammography and should not be used alone to detect breast cancer. Sometimes it is helpful in interpreting mammography.

HYSTERECTOMY AND SURGICAL MENOPAUSE

Hysterectomy is the surgical removal of a woman's uterus. Once you have a hysterectomy you will not menstruate and cannot become pregnant. When one or both of your ovaries are left in, the surgery does not lead to an immediate menopause. Cyclic hormonal changes continue every month, even though you do not get periods.

Why Are They Done?

"I'll tell you, the last months before the surgery I was so sick, suffering so much, that I was fine when it was all over. I had no more pain, and everything went well."

The three most common conditions leading to hysterectomy in North America are fibroids, heavy bleeding and pelvic relaxation (see page 109). Not everyone agrees as to when hysterectomy is appropriate. The following are some common situations in which it is done.

Large Fibroids. Fibroids, the most common reason for hysterectomy in North America, are benign tumors in the muscle of the uterus.

Some fibroids can be removed surgically without removing the uterus. You may have to shop around for a doctor who is willing to do this. In deciding for or against hysterectomy you need to consider the severity of your symptoms as well as your age. Because the growth of fibroids is stimulated by estrogen, they shrink after menopause. If you are close to menopause you may choose to wait. If not, and your symptoms are severe, you may find waiting impossible.

Abnormal Bleeding. Heavy and/or irregular bleeding which do not respond to curettage (D & C, pages 101-4), or progesterone therapy (page 54) is a common reason for hysterectomy. As with fibroids, the problem ends with menopause, so your age enters into the decision-making.

Pelvic Relaxation. Sometimes the muscles of the pelvic floor stretch, allowing the pelvic organs to descend and bulge into the vagina . Although this is a common reason for hysterectomy, other measures can be taken and hysterectomy should be a last resort. Kegel exercises (page 111) are useful for both prevention and treatment of pelvic relaxation. A pessary (a device similar to a diaphragm, which is worn in the vagina) can be used to support a descending uterus and surgical procedures other than hysterectomy do exist.

Cancer. Cancer can affect the uterus at three sites: the cervix, the endometrium and the muscle.

Cancer of the cervix has decreased dramatically since the introduction of the Pap test, a simple procedure which detects pre-cancerous cells. Abnormal cells are destroyed either with cryosurgery (freezing) or with a laser beam. Hysterectomy is used only in advanced cases or when other problems co-exist.

Cancer of the endometrium is a growth of cancerous cells in the lining of the uterus. Most common in post-menopausal women, it is linked to high estrogen levels, obesity and high blood pressure.

Cancer of the uterine muscle is very rare.

Extensive Endometriosis. In this condition, endometrial tissue grows outside the uterus and bleeds cyclically each month, causing considerable pain and scarring. If you are nearing menopause you may decide to wait and see if your symptoms

HYSTERECTOMY

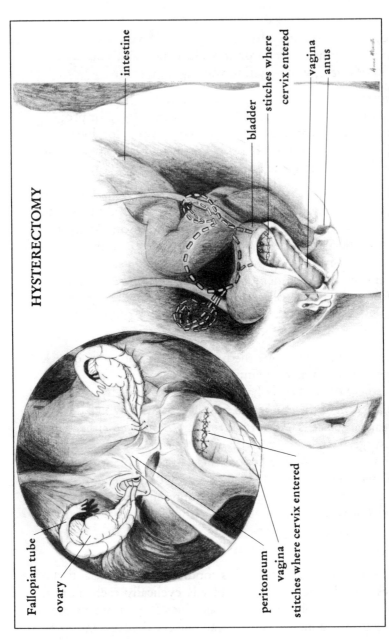

intestine

bladder

stitches where cervix entered

vagina

anus

Fallopian tube

ovary

peritoneum

vagina

stitches where cervix entered

After hysterectomy. Uterus with cervix, ovaries and fallopian tubes removed. Inset: Only uterus with cervix removed. The peritoneum (membrane lining the abdominal cavity) is stitched after removal of the uterus.

KEGEL EXERCISES

The pelvic floor muscles hold the pelvic organs — the uterus, bladder and rectum — in place in the pelvis. Childbirth can weaken these muscles and result in these organs bulging or dropping down into the vagina (prolapse). This may cause pain, a feeling of heaviness in the pelvic area or stress incontinence. Stress incontinence is the leaking of urine when you cough, sneeze, laugh or do certain physical activities. Pelvic floor relaxation is one of the most common reasons why hysterectomy is performed.

Kegel exercises strengthen pelvic muscles and help to prevent prolapse. They are also extremely useful immediately after childbirth to help tighten up the pelvic floor muscles and prevent later problems.

Kegel exercises are done as follows:

1. First find the pelvic floor muscles that you will be exercising by starting and stopping the flow of urine. The muscles you use to stop the flow are the right ones.
2. Contract (tighten) these muscles for a second or two, then relax them. That is the Kegel exercise.
3. Start by doing 10 Kegels, and work up to about 5 - 7 minutes a day. They don't all have to be done at once. You can do them at any time — reading, on the bus, driving to work, as part of your regular exercise routine.

are relieved once your periods stop. Younger women in severe pain from extensive endometriosis may opt for hysterectomy.

Severe Chronic Pelvic Inflammatory Disease (PID). Pelvic infections are usually caused by sexually transmitted diseases such as gonorrhea or chlamydia, and are more common with IUD use. Chronic PID which causes severe pain that cannot be relieved by other treatments is sometimes treated with hysterectomy.

Hysterectomy is particularly controversial in two situations: sterilization and cancer prevention.

Sterilization. In the past, tubal ligations were restricted to women with many children or those with serious health problems. When other birth control methods were ineffective or unacceptable, women and their doctors sometimes exaggerated medical problems to justify a hysterectomy, when what they really wanted was sterilization. Today tubal ligation is more widely available. It is a safer and cheaper method of sterilization and maintains the uterus intact.

Hysterectomies are sometimes performed to stop menstruation in women who have certain types of psychosis and fear of blood or women who are severely retarded or unable to take care of themselves. Recently in Quebec, a human rights group prevented a couple from having a hysterectomy performed on their mentally handicapped daughter. The parents argued that their daughter had a phobic loathing of blood and was incapable of coping with her periods. The human rights group presented arguments against unnecessary surgery and in favor of the right of all women to normal bodily functions. The balance between respecting a disabled person's rights and the practical aspects of chronic care is a delicate one. The history of past abuse has led the courts to be extremely prudent in cases of involuntary sterilization.

Cancer Prevention. Cancer prevention is not considered an acceptable reason for hysterectomy on its own. However, when a woman has a minor medical problem or wants to be sterilized, she is often convinced to have a hysterectomy based on the rationale of preventing endometrial cancer. Fear of cancer is also used to justify the removal of healthy ovaries at the time of a hysterectomy.

"I had a total. The doctor said if I had been younger she would have done a partial, but because it's usually the ovaries that get cancerous it was total."

Types of Surgery

Several types of hysterectomy are possible. The extent of surgery (which organs are removed) is determined by the medical condition and the desire to prevent cancer.

Total/Complete hysterectomy involves the removal of the uterus including the cervix. The place in the vagina where the cervix used to enter is sewn together. This is the most commonly performed procedure today.

Sub-total hysterectomy involves removal of the body of the uterus only; the cervix and vagina are left intact. This type of hysterectomy was common before antibiotics, when opening the vagina greatly increased the risk of infection. In this era of antibiotics and improved surgical technique, gynecologists routinely remove the cervix, thus eliminating a possible focus for cancer. Some doctors and health groups are now questioning whether leaving the cervix would reduce the negative effect of hysterectomy on sexuality (see page 117). Pap tests reduce the risk of cervical cancer. It is hard to know whether this type of hysterectomy is advantageous since it has been performed so rarely over the past 25 years.

Radical hysterectomy refers to removal of the body of the uterus including the cervix, as well as the upper part of the vagina and the surrounding lymph nodes. Radical hysterectomy is used when the spread of cancer is suspected.

Total hysterectomy and bilateral salpingo-ovariectomy is the removal of the uterus, cervix, Fallopian tubes and both ovaries. This is the usual treatment of a condition affecting both the uterus and ovaries. It is often recommended to middle-aged women, even with healthy ovaries, as a method of preventing ovarian cancer.

Hysterectomy is performed through an incision either in the abdomen or upper vagina. Abdominal hysterectomy is used when the abdomen or pelvis must be explored to help make a diagnosis; when there are signs of pelvic infection;

when the uterus is very large; when a woman has had prior pelvic surgery including a cesarean delivery; or when the ovaries must also be removed. The incision is made either horizontally along the pubic line (bikini cut) or vertically from below the navel to the pubic bone. The horizontal incision heals faster and is less noticeable afterwards.

Vaginal hysterectomy is done in cases of prolapsed uterus, or when a bladder repair to treat stress incontinence (leakage of urine from the bladder) is done at the same time. The risk of major complications can be lower with vaginal hysterectomy if the surgeon is experienced doing this particular surgical technique. The healing time is also shorter.

Effects of Surgery

"A few days after the surgery, when the drugs were really wearing off, I noticed that I was getting hot — very hot — and I asked the nurse if it's normal and she got the doctor and he told me that now, without my ovaries I was in my menopause. I thought he was kidding me at first. Well I was surprised and a bit embarassed and then I was a bit angry that he hadn't told me. But it wouldn't have changed anything."

Short-Term Effects. During the immediate recovery period you will have some pain and be very tired. You may be weepy, especially during the week in the hospital, and may experience hot flashes for a short period even if your ovaries have not been removed.

The majority of short-term complications are similar to the risks of other abdominal surgery. Anesthetic risks are greater if you have breathing difficulties such as asthma, are a heavy smoker or have many allergies.

Hemorrhage can occur during surgery, and less likely,

afterwards. If you lose a great deal of blood, a transfusion may be necessary. Otherwise you need to take iron tablets for a few months to replenish your red blood cells.

During surgery, injury can occur to the organs near your uterus including the bladder, ureters (tubes leading from each kidney to the bladder) and bowel.

"A long time after my hysterectomy, when it was time for my period, I'd have cramps in my abdomen, the same as if I was going to have my period. Like the day before. I don't know if it was in my mind, but the day before I used to have cramps, the same as if I was going to get my period."

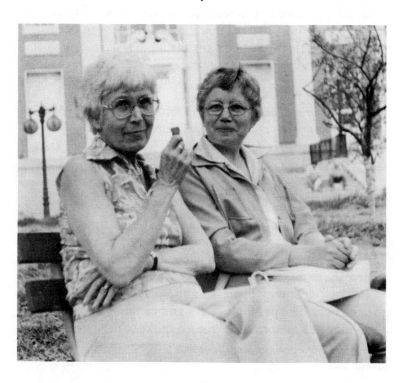

Long-Term Effects. A hysterectomy usually has some psychological impact — sometimes positive, sometimes negative. Many women feel relieved, physically better and more energetic after their hysterectomy. This is especially true for women who had a difficult time before the surgery and find themselves suddenly relieved of painful and disruptive symptoms and for women with cancer, whose lives may be saved by the surgery.

"After the hysterectomy I felt a thousand times better. Much more female. I felt so good about me. Certainly much more sexual."

If pain or bleeding interfered with your sex life before your hysterectomy, there should be a big improvement afterward. The fact that unplanned pregnancy is no longer a worry may also give your sex life a boost.

"It was such a delicious feeling to know I was never going to have another period, and no matter what I do, I can never become pregnant again."

But more women become depressed after hysterectomy than after other major surgery. The depression can start months after the surgery, so that often the gynecologist never finds out about it. This partly explains why doctors may not warn women about it.

It is not clear why depression should be so common after hysterectomy. The psychological significance of the loss of the uterus may be a factor. Some women spoke to us of a profound sorrow at their inability to have children (even if they had no plans to have any more). Others spoke of feeling scarred, unattractive, no longer a complete woman. There may be physical or hormonal explanations for depression. Regardless of the cause, it is important to know that depression is a real possibility after hysterectomy and to recognize that it is not a personal failing. Ways of handling depression are discussed on page 90.

Some of us experience other long-term consequences of hysterectomy and ovariectomy for which we are often not prepared. For example, many women experience a decreased sexual response, particularly if they have had their ovaries removed.

A commonly held belief both in the medical and lay communities is that sexual problems after hysterectomy are in your head. Yet new studies are now confirming that the physical effects of hysterectomy and ovariectomy may contribute to the sexual changes that some of us experience.

Some women miss the sensations caused by the rising up of their uterus into the pelvis during the excitement phase. The vaginal scar sometimes causes pain with intercourse. Some women find orgasm is different and sometimes less intense after the surgery, possibly because they no longer have rhythmic uterine contractions during orgasm. Some women find orgasm difficult to achieve if their cervix is not stimulated during sexual activity. They may especially notice a difference in orgasm brought on by deep penetration since that is the kind of sexual activity that would have previously stimulated their cervix.

Women who have had their ovaries removed often have the greatest difficulty sexually. The ovaries produce androgens, hormones which are believed to affect libido (sex drive). After surgery, with fewer androgens, a woman may notice a drop in her sexual desire. Some doctors recommend androgen therapy for women who have had their ovaries removed (see page 124).

Estrogen, also produced by the ovaries, keeps the tissues of the vagina lush and helps the vagina to lubricate during arousal. Ovariectomy can lead to decreased lubrication and fragile vaginal tissue which can make intercourse painful. (See Part 2 – Vaginal Changes.)

Young women whose ovaries are removed have a higher risk of developing heart disease than other women their age. The younger the woman is at the time of surgery, the greater the risk for heart disease. In women with no other risk factors, HRT seems to reduce this risk. Some research shows an increase in heart disease even if only the uterus has been removed. The reason for this is not understood.

"The doctor said 'you are young, and you can not live without hormones.' So since the age of 26 I've been taking hormones: Premarin."

Although not all studies agree, some evidence suggests that hysterectomy brings on a slightly earlier menopause, even when a woman's ovaries are not removed. Some women gain weight after hysterectomy just as many do after menopause. The cause may be metabolic; that is, the rate at which we burn off calories may slow down. Some of us become more sedentary after surgery, while others may unknowingly eat more. After ovariectomy, hormonal changes may also explain weight gain.

SURGICAL MENOPAUSE – OVARIECTOMY

Ovariectomy (oophorectomy) is the surgical removal of an ovary. When one ovary is removed before menopause, the remaining ovary produces enough hormones to maintain the menstrual cycle. Menopause occurs at the same age or only slightly earlier.

When both ovaries are removed (bilateral ovariectomy), you experience instantaneous menopause or female castration. It is equivalent to removing a man's testicles. After surgery, hormone levels drop to post-menopausal levels within hours. Bilateral ovariectomy prior to menopause creates a sudden, artificial menopause. Hot flashes and other symptoms may be severe and women often begin hormone replacement therapy immediately after surgery. If you have already been through menopause when your ovaries are removed, you will not experience the same dramatic drop in hormone levels that pre-menopausal women do.

Women who undergo ovariectomy prior to menopause experience an early decrease in bone density. Because these women spend more years without the protective effect of estrogen, they have a greater chance of developing osteoporosis (page 77).

A number of conditions dictate removal of the ovaries, including ovarian cancer, benign ovarian cysts which can rupture or press on other organs causing pain, severe pelvic inflammatory disease or extensive endometriosis affecting the ovaries. Women with certain types of breast cancer are sometimes counselled to have their ovaries removed to reduce the stimulation of the cancer cells by estrogen.

The big debate surrounding ovariectomy centres on the removal of healthy ovaries to prevent ovarian cancer. Ovarian cancer rates are relatively low compared with other kinds of reproductive organ cancers. However no effective screening test exists for ovarian cancer similar to the Pap test for cervical cancer. Because detection is difficult, it often is not discovered until well advanced and difficult to treat. This leads some doctors to suggest that all women have their ovaries removed "while they're in there" doing a hysterectomy. With increasing understanding of the important role of estrogen in

119

preventing osteoporosis, the practice now is not to remove the healthy ovaries of women under 40.

More and more evidence shows that the ovaries still serve a function in post-menopausal women. They continue to produce estrogen for years after menopause and they are the main source of androgens, hormones believed to be important to libido (sex drive). An increasingly vocal group of doctors, researchers and women believe that, except in unique circumstances such as a strong family history of ovarian cancer, healthy ovaries should not be removed. The removal of any healthy organ is questionable medical practice. The rationale for such a decision should be clearly stated and the consequences well understood.

Making The Decision

Unfortunately, in most cases making a decision about hysterectomy and ovariectomy is difficult, complex and far from absolute.

Knowing the answers to a few questions in particular would be very useful, but you cannot answer them without a crystal ball. It would help to know, for example, at what age you will go through menopause. Flooding might be tolerable if you knew it would be over in a few months. If endometrial or ovarian cancer is in your future, the decision would be more clear cut as well.

As with other decisions about your body, the final decision should be yours alone since you must live with the consequences, both good and bad. But you need, and should get, plenty of help with the decision. A primary source of help is a doctor who will clearly explain the medical implications of both your condition and the surgery. We strongly recommend that you get a second opinion as well, preferably from a doctor not affiliated with your own. If the second doctor agrees that surgery is necessary, you can be that much more confident of your decision to go ahead. If the two doctors disagree, you will have heard the case presented for and against surgery in your situation and you will be better equipped to make your decision.

Other women who have had a similar experience are excellent sources of information and advice.

"One day at a checkup he asked my age and I was 43 or 45. He asked if I wanted any more children. I said certainly not so he said why don't we get it out? Have a hysterectomy. I asked if I really needed it and he said,

---

THE POLITICS OF HYSTERECTOMY

Although hysterectomy rates have declined slightly in the past ten years, hysterectomy is still the most common major operation in North America today. At present, close to sixty percent of us will have our uterus removed by the age of sixty.

Hysterectomy rates vary depending on where you live and your socio-economic status. For example, rates are much higher in the Atlantic provinces than in the rest of Canada. In the United States, women with health insurance have twice as many hysterectomies as those without. Also, higher hysterectomy rates exist in countries where doctors are paid per operation than in those where doctors are salaried. These astounding statistics have led health practitioners and consumers alike to question the number of hysterectomies performed.

Certain attitudes contribute to the hysterectomy rate. For example, once childbearing is complete, the uterus is considered by some to be a useless, disease-prone organ and periods are seen as a nuisance we would all be better off without. This philosophy ignores the growing evidence that the uterus has other roles beyond carrying babies, especially with regard to sexuality. It also goes against the recent trend to avoid removing organs unnecessarily — such as tonsils — because they may have multiple purposes, including some of which we may not be aware.

"Look, you don't need the organ anymore. Take it out." I asked "Would you take my tonsils out too?" He said, 'Come on. Either you trust me or you don't.'"

❖

Some questions to ask yourself in thinking this decision through include: How bad are your symptoms? Can you live with them, and if so for how long? Will menopause relieve your condition? How old are you and what is your menopausal status? Are there any long-term risks to your health from this condition? What risk factors do you have for endometrial cancer, ovarian cancer and osteoporosis? How do you feel about the possibility of having to take hormones?

Take your time in answering these questions and reflecting on the answers. You can and should go home and think about the decision. Except in the case of an emergency, you do not have to make the decision in the doctor's office. Most important, any discussion, questioning and decision-making should happen before you are admitted to the hospital. Most of us feel helpless in the hospital setting. We are often stressed, and without the people who usually support us. A hospital bed on the night before surgery is not the place to make a decision about whether to have your ovaries removed or whether to have a hysterectomy at all.

HORMONE REPLACEMENT THERAPY

"The word hormone scares the heck out of me. I like things to be as natural as possible. So for as long as possible I would like to go along, until the point where if it becomes unbearable, then I will broach the subject. Right now I'm not interested."

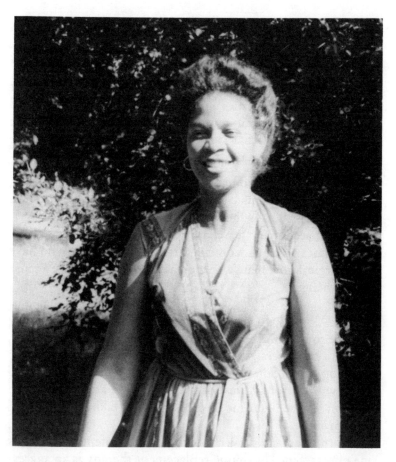

In hormone replacement therapy, natural or synthetic (artificial) hormones are used to relieve uncomfortable symptoms associated with menopause, to prevent osteoporosis, or both. At first, when only estrogen was used, the treatment was called estrogen replacement therapy (ERT). Hormone replacement therapy (HRT) refers to treatment combining any of the following hormones:

Estrogen comes in natural (e.g. conjugated estrogen) or

synthetic (e.g. ethinyl estradiol) form. Natural estrogen, used most commonly, is best known under the brand name Premarin. Estrogen relieves many symptoms of menopause.

Progesterone is used in pill form together with estrogen or occasionally alone as an injection. It has been incorporated into hormone therapy in recent years in an attempt to decrease the risk of endometrial cancer (cancer of the lining of the uterus) associated with estrogen.

Testosterone is a hormone produced by both men and women, but in greater amounts by men. One of a group of hormones called androgens, it is the hormone responsible for the development of secondary sex characteristics in men. Testosterone is sometimes given to women, particularly to those who have had a surgical menopause, to increase sex drive and give a sense of well-being.

Traditionally doctors recommended HRT as a temporary measure to help women over a difficult period. More recently, medical researchers are encouraging its use for the prevention of osteoporosis. Some go so far as to propose the use of HRT for all women for the rest of their lives. We are beginning to envision for the first time the possibility of taking HRT for 30 years or more.

Hormones are powerful drugs with potentially serious side effects. Since hormone replacement therapy is an aggressive approach to the changes that sometimes accompany menopause, we need to be very sure that the benefits of treatment outweigh the risks.

Historical and Social Context

Use of estrogens in modern medicine began in the 1930s with the discovery of DES, the first synthetic estrogen. Within months, before any long-term safety testing was done, it was on the market. Its disastrous consequences were known only

30 years later, when the children of the women who took it began developing health problems.

By the 1970s estrogen was one of the five most prescribed drugs in the U.S., earning approximately $70 million a year in profits for the drug companies. A large portion of these sales came from the birth control pill, but estrogen treatment was also popular for treating depression, anxiety and hot flashes in mid-life women, and for "preventing" aging.

In 1947, a warning was sounded in the medical journals about a possible link between estrogen replacement therapy and cancer of the lining of the uterus. Yet it was not until 1975 that the first serious studies were published showing a significant increase of this kind of cancer in women taking estrogen. Reports in the popular media followed, causing a great deal of concern. Many women stopped taking estrogen.

What is the situation now, in the 1990s, with hormone replacement therapy? As the baby boom generation ages, menopause is receiving a great deal more attention. Awareness of osteoporosis as a major health problem and promotion of the long-term use of HRT to prevent it are both increasing.

Drug companies are taking advantage of this concern about osteoporosis to improve the image of hormone therapy and thus increase sales. Their focus has shifted from hormones as treatment for short-term discomforts to hormones as a solution to a chronic health problem. They are promoting hormones as an essential part of a program of health maintenance for mid-life and older women. So far, in spite of their efforts, the majority of women still do not take HRT.

The generation approaching menopause in the 1990s has lived through a number of drug catastrophes. We have seen the deformed limbs of children whose mothers took thalidomide during pregnancy. We also experienced the far-reaching effects on the health and fertility of children whose mothers took DES to prevent miscarriage. We may be more wary of new drugs and of untested new uses for old drugs. We are also a

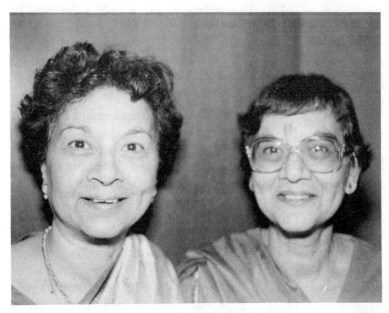

generation which has seen a proliferation of alternative health care providers and settings, with some very promising, others just as profit-oriented and power-hungry as the traditional health care system can be. We may be more comfortable going beyond traditional medicine and medications in our search for solutions. Some of us have access to more information and are in a better position to make informed decisions about what is best for us.

Making The Decision

HRT is a very controversial issue in women's health, with people in extreme camps ranging from "estrogen for every woman for life" to "estrogen for no woman" regardless of the severity of her problems.

Looking at social and medical attitudes towards women and menopause, the historical context in which hormones have been used, as well as the interests of special groups like the drug companies, is part of coming to a decision. So is understanding the biological process of menopause and the effects of the hormones.

Responsible health care workers face conflicts about what recommendations to make. This makes it even more difficult for us to decide whether or not to take hormone replacement therapy, when and for how long.

Ultimately the decision whether or not to take hormones rests with you; you are the one reaping the benefits but also taking the risks. This is a personal decision which must be made with the knowledge that all the information is not yet in. For instance, who will develop complications from hormones? Who is likely to develop endometrial cancer? Are we among the 25% of women who will suffer fractures due to severe osteoporosis? Consider your personal health history, your lifestyle and values. Most important, assess how difficult you are finding your menopausal symptoms and how concerned you are about osteoporosis.

Your decision does not have to be made in the doctor's office. Take your time. Take weeks or even months to decide if necessary. Be clear on the reasons for your decision and plan to reevaluate regularly. The factors upon which you based your original decision may change. Try to avoid feeling pressured or guilty. And there is no point in our judging each other's choices since there is no right answer for everyone.

The rest of this section deals with the specifics of HRT: what it treats, what it doesn't treat, its side effects and how to take it.

"The doctor told me about hormones. He gave me 3 articles. One was very favourable to hormones, one was not as favourable and one article was very anti-hormones.

They were from reputable medical journals yet they were very different. He told me to read them and then he would answer any questions I might have. I did read them, and I decided that hormones weren't for me. I think if my symptoms had been severe I might have had a different response and requested hormones."

What It Can Do
Hormone replacement therapy has several proven benefits.
Hot Flashes. HRT provides complete and rapid relief from hot flashes. When prescribed only to treat flashes, take the lowest dose that works, for the shortest period of time possible.

When you go off the hormones abruptly, hot flashes often return for a while. This is true no matter how many years after menopause you stop the medication. This means that you can postpone hot flashes but there is no guarantee that you can completely avoid them unless you take the hormones for the rest of your life. You may prevent or diminish this rebound effect by slowly weaning yourself from the hormones rather than stopping suddenly.

Depo-Provera, a controversial drug used for birth control, is not recommended for use at menopause, but is sometimes prescribed for women with hot flashes who feel they need to take medication but cannot take estrogen. Less effective than estrogen, it probably carries more health risks.

Vaginal Changes. Painful thinning of the vaginal walls together with decreased lubrication sometimes causes problems after menopause. HRT can help by reversing these changes. Although not permanent, the reversal sometimes lasts for months. Therefore some women can take hormones for a few months and then be off them for months or even a year.

Estrogen for vaginal changes is often prescribed in the form of a vaginal cream. Many women do not realize that the hormones in vaginal creams are absorbed into the bloodstream just as pills are, and have all of the same side effects. If you take estrogen creams for more than one or two months, you should also take progesterone pills for the last 10 days of treatment just as if you were taking estrogen by mouth. This is to reduce the risk of endometrial cancer. Progesterone itself has no effect on vaginal changes.

Osteoporosis. Growing evidence shows that estrogen prevents the bone changes of osteoporosis by decreasing bone breakdown (resorption). When combined with calcium and an exercise program, HRT may even increase bone mass. HRT does seem to relieve some of the bone pain of osteoporosis.

"My mother was on Premarin and then was taken off, and she says her bones ache. When she was left on it she felt fine."

There is much debate about how exactly the hormones act to prevent bone loss. Do they increase bone mass or simply prevent mineral loss? Can they prevent fractures? Are they useful for women who already have osteoporosis? What happens if you stop? Since bone loss accelerates quickly in the first few years after menopause, the sooner you start the treatment, the more positive the effects.

As long as the treatment continues bone loss seems to slow down, but when treatment is stopped bone loss resumes and may actually accelerate. Whether it accelerates is a key question; the answer will influence how long HRT should be taken. If bone loss increased gradually, it would seem reasonable for a woman to stop HRT after a certain number of years, confident that she had pushed back the age at which she would risk fracturing bones. If, on the other hand, bone loss is rapid after stopping HRT, a woman who starts it should probably continue it for life. As yet we do not know the answer. We have absolutely no idea what the effects of such long-term use of hormones will be. The women now on such an osteoporosis prevention program are in effect guinea pigs in a large experiment. We are learning about any good or bad effects of long-term hormone use by watching what happens to them.

Taking calcium with estrogen probably increases its effectiveness and may decrease the dose of estrogen needed.

Progesterone alone does not seem to have the same protective effect on bone as estrogen except at unacceptably high doses.

Heart Disease. Since estrogen is known to have a good

DEPO-PROVERA

Depo-Provera (Medroxyprogesterone acetate) is a long-lasting synthetic form of progesterone, given by injection every three months. Although most famous as a birth control method, some doctors and textbooks recommend it for treatment of hot flashes.

Depo-Provera was developed in the United States as a treatment for endometriosis and to prevent miscarriage. In Canada it is approved only for treatment of endometriosis and to relieve pain in certain types of cancer. Nevertheless, doctors prescribe it for birth control and to treat hot flashes in women who cannot take estrogen. It is difficult to determine the number of women actually using it for these purposes.

In spite of heavy lobbying, the drug company which produces Depo-Provera has been unable to have it approved for contraceptive use in the United States. In Canada the lobbying has been more effective. The government is leaning towards approving it for birth control, and refusing to hold open hearings to hear the many objections to this drug.

The known side effects of Depo-Provera include nausea, depression, weight gain or loss, decreased interest in sex, breakthrough bleeding, breast tenderness and prolonged absence of menstruation.

(continued)

effect on the fat in the blood (including cholesterol), it is believed to protect against heart disease. Because a woman's chances of having a heart attack go up after menopause, experts are promoting HRT to reduce heart disease in post-menopausal women.

So far, this benefit has only been proven in women who had their ovaries removed before menopause. Whether or not it also applies to women who go through a natural menopause is under study but not yet proven.

The issue of taking HRT to prevent heart disease is confused by the effect of progesterone on fat in the blood. Unlike estrogen, it is known to have a bad effect on the fat in the blood (including cholesterol), and therefore may increase the risk of

---

(continued)

The controversy which surrounds the drug is not over these side effects, but over possible long-term complications including infertility, breast cancer and endometrial cancer.

Proponents of Depo-Provera claim that the animals chosen for research are especially prone to breast cancer. They believe the drug is relatively safe, particularly when weighed against the high infant and maternal mortality rates in many of the countries where it is used. Some of the biggest supporters of Depo-Provera are individuals and agencies whose primary interest is in population control, particularly in the Third World, rather than in the health or contraceptive needs of individual women. Some women who use it like the simplicity of an injection every three months.

Opponents of Depo-Provera feel that at best the results of animal studies are inconclusive. Since there appear to be such potentially serious risks, they feel women should not be the guinea pigs upon whom the conclusive research is done. They are also concerned that many women, particularly those in Third World countries, are not given all the information they need to make an informed choice.

Provera, the pill form of medroxyprogesterone acetate, is commonly used for the progesterone portion of HRT. The controversy over Depo-Provera does not apply to Provera.

---

heart disease. This might undo the benefits of the estrogen.

More research is needed to determine whether estrogen treatment does have benefits for heart disease and whether those benefits remain after adding progesterone as is generally recommended in HRT.

What It Probably Cannot Do

In spite of the promises of the 1960s, estrogen is not the fountain of youth. No drug has been found which stops or turns back the normal aging progress.

Estrogen affects the skin by increasing its thickness, but it does not prevent wrinkles. Genetics and prior sun exposure are important determinants of wrinkling.

Whether estrogen has an effect on menopausal changes other than "the big four" is unclear. Some studies have shown estrogen to relieve depression and anxiety, possibly by affecting certain chemicals in the brain. Other studies show no such improvement. Any effect on mood may be due to the relief of hot flashes and sleep disruption or possibly to the improvement in vaginal changes and therefore in sexual pleasure.

There are similar questions about the effect of estrogen on insomnia (sleeplessness or severely disturbed sleep patterns). Estrogen may have a chemical effect on the brain which improves sleep patterns. It does eliminate hot flashes which may waken you. Flashes which are not quite strong enough to wake you up completely may nonetheless disturb your sleep, so controlling the flashes with estrogen may restore restful sleep.

Sometimes tranquilizers are included in estrogen pills, with or without the knowledge of the woman taking them. Relief of anxiety and depression probably results from the hidden tranquilizers and not the hormones. Based on what we know so far, it is wrong to use hormones as if they were antidepressants or tranquilizers.

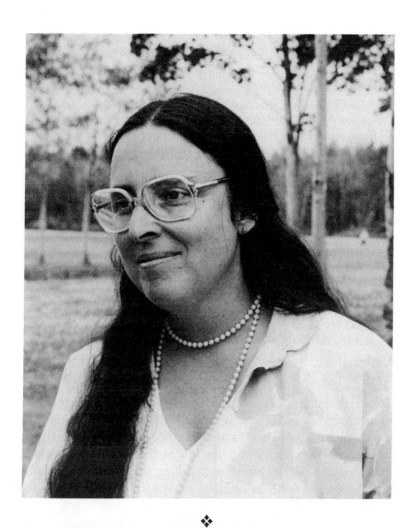

❖

*"I started a few days after surgery, and I have no more
hot flashes, but I never had any other symptoms. They
haven't made me feel my own age though. I feel older
than my age. They haven't really made me feel more
sexual desire."*

❖

HIDDEN TRANQUILIZERS

The widespread use of tranquilizers has had an enormous effect on the lives and health of women. Women are consistently prescribed more mood-altering drugs than men at every stage of life. As women age, they use these drugs even more frequently. Although tranquilizers have a definite role in situations of acute anxiety, they have long been used as medical band-aids for social problems such as poverty, loneliness and bad relationships. Women often seek out and continue to take these drugs because without them their situations seem intolerable and because they are not supported or encouraged to find long term-solutions.

Tranquilizers produce serious side effects and can be addictive. When they are hidden inside other medications, we are not aware of what we are taking or what the possible side effects may be.

Certain preparations of estrogen available for HRT contain tranquilizers. Menrium, available in both the U.S. and Canada, contains Chlordiazepoxide (Librium) and estrified estrogens. Often women are not told precisely what is being prescribed for them, and it may not be evident from the label. We find this practice unacceptable and encourage women to verify their prescriptions.

The Risks

In weighing the decision to use any kind of medication, take two kinds of side effects into account: dangerous complications, and effects that are a nuisance but not dangerous. If you have major complications from taking the hormones, you will have to stop. If you experience minor side effects, you must decide whether the benefits of the treatment are worth the inconveniences.

Nuisance side effects known to be associated with hormone therapy include withdrawal bleeding, breast tenderness, leg cramps and increased body hair (with androgen therapy only). There may be other side effects that we do not yet know about.

Withdrawal Bleeding. This happens when you go off the hormones between days 26 and 30. (see How To Take It, page 141).

Withdrawal bleeding is not a dangerous sign. In fact, it is advantageous because it allows the endometrium to thin out. Usually this withdrawal bleeding stops after a few months or a year of treatment. Many women see withdrawal bleeding as the return of their periods and consider it a drawback to taking HRT.

The amount of bleeding you have is affected by the amount of estrogen you are taking. The lower the dose, the less frequently this side effect occurs. If you are taking progesterone as well as estrogen, the bleeding will often occur every month like a light period.

Breast Tenderness. You may experience breast tenderness with estrogen, particularly if you are taking high doses. Lowering the dose, for example from 1.25 to .625 mg, may eliminate the problem. Progesterone does not have any effect on breast tenderness.

Leg Cramps. Some women experience leg cramps which can be a side effect of either estrogen or progesterone. Why estrogen causes leg cramps is not well understood. Progesterone's effect is probably due to the dilatation (widening) of the veins in the legs or possibly to fluid retention. Lowering the dose of hormone may decrease the cramps. If the pain is in one leg only and accompanied by swelling and redness, you should be examined to be sure it is not caused by a blood clot.

Increased Body Hair. This is a possible side effect of testosterone which is sometimes given together with estrogen.

Serious complications associated with hormone therapy include mid-cycle or breakthrough bleeding, endometrial cancer, gallstones and, possibly, recurrence of fibroids and endometriosis.

Mid-Cycle Bleeding. This type of bleeding occurs while you are taking estrogen. It is usually due to endometrial hyperplasia, an overgrowth of the cells of the lining of the uterus.

Mid-cycle vaginal bleeding can also be a sign of endometrial cancer. It is always important to determine why you are having mid-cycle bleeding.

Endometrial Cancer. Estrogen therapy alone greatly increases your risk of developing cancer of the endometrium. The higher the dosage the greater the risk, and the longer you take estrogen without progesterone, the greater the risk.

Taking progesterone for 10 days each month along with the estrogen reverses endometrial overgrowth (hyperplasia) and strong evidence suggests that it reduces the risk of developing endometrial cancer. However this drug regimen — HRT as opposed to ERT — is still relatively new. As with the long-term use of estrogen, those of us taking it are, in effect, part of an experiment, the results of which are not yet known.

The risk of endometrial cancer is increased for women who are overweight, who have high blood pressure or endometrial hyperplasia, or those who have never had a baby. Women with these risk factors need closer follow-up if they do decide to take hormones.

While not minimizing its effect on women's lives, we should point out that endometrial cancer is an illness for which treatment is very often successful, particularly for post-menopausal women.

Gallstones. Women who take HRT run a greater risk of devel-

RISK FACTORS FOR ENDOMETRIAL CANCER

- obesity
- diabetes
- high blood pressure
- infrequent ovulation due to hormone imbalance
- use of estrogen other than in birth control pill*

* some studies show that taking the birth control pill actually reduces the risk of endometrial and ovarian cancer.

---

oping gallstones. Estrogen taken in pill form passes through the liver and affects the function of both the liver and gallbladder. Estrogens taken by other routes (see insert) have much less effect because they are absorbed directly into the bloodstream without first passing through the liver. If you are overweight, you are already at higher risk for gallstones and should take that into account when considering HRT.

Fibroids. Fibroids, benign tumors in the muscle of the uterus, depend on estrogen for their growth, and therefore shrink after menopause. HRT reintroduces the estrogen and the possibility that the fibroids will grow again. With low doses of estrogen, this does not seem to be a problem.

Endometriosis. Although reports of HRT causing a recurrence are few, the Endometriosis Society of Canada suggests that women who had severe endometriosis before menopause use HRT cautiously.

Other side effects may exist that we do not yet know about. There are also some health concerns surrounding HRT which have not yet proved to be problems, but which are still being investigated.

High Blood Pressure. The increased risk of developing high

RISK FACTORS FOR BREAST CANCER

- over 50 years old*
- family history (mother, sister) of breast cancer before menopause, especially if family member had cancer in both breasts*
- previous breast cancer*
- certain fibrocystic breast conditions
- high fat diet
- first period before age 12
- late menopause
- no pregnancies

* *highest risk*

---

blood pressure with birth control pills has caused concern about the relationship between blood pressure and HRT. The risk of developing high blood pressure depends on how much hormone you take. The lower estrogen doses used in HRT pose less of a problem. Still, many doctors try to avoid HRT in women with high blood pressure.

Breast Cancer. This has been an area of constant concern since hormones were first marketed. Until recently research did not link estrogen to breast cancer. However studies suggest that under certain circumstances, the rate of breast cancer may increase in women taking hormones, either in the birth control pill or in HRT. Particularly unsettling is a recent study which found that progesterone, which was added to HRT to protect against endometrial cancer, may actually increase the risk of breast cancer.

These findings are not yet having an effect on the prescription of hormones to women. The consensus seems to be that it is still too early to draw firm conclusions about the links between hormones and breast cancer. However, there are those who feel that women already at high risk of developing breast cancer would do well to act with caution until more is known. We need to insist that more research be done to clarify this important issue for all women.

Certain types of breast cancer are known to grow more quickly when stimulated by estrogen. If you develop that kind of cancer, tumour growth will increase with the added estro-

---

RISK FACTORS FOR OVARIAN CANCER

- family history of ovarian cancer, breast cancer
- never had children
- history of extensive exposure of pelvis to radiation
- use of estrogen other than in birth control pill*

* *some studies show that taking the birth control pill actually reduces the risk of endometrial and ovarian cancer*

---

gen in HRT. This is a particular concern for women at high risk of developing breast cancer.

Heart Disease and Stroke. The increased risk of heart disease and stroke among women taking the birth control pill has caused some concern about HRT. However estrogen and progesterone at the doses they are given to menopausal women appear not to increase the risk of developing heart disease and stroke. The amount of hormone in HRT is approximately 10 times less than that used in the average birth control pill, which may explain the difference in side effects.

When To Start

Many women wonder when the right time is to start hormones. This depends on why you are taking them. If you are using the hormone replacement therapy to treat symptoms, there is no point in starting before you actually have symptoms to treat. If the symptoms never come, or if they are not troublesome when they do come, then you may never need to start. This is

---

CONTRAINDICATIONS TO HRT

If you have the following conditions you should not take HRT:

1. estrogen-dependent cancers (some types of breast and kidney cancer)
2. severe or chronic liver disease
3. a history of blood clots or inflammation of veins in the legs
4. vaginal bleeding for which a reason has not yet been found

If you have the following conditions you should carefully consider your special risk factors before taking HRT:

1. fibroids
2. high blood cholesterol
3. high blood pressure
4. severe varicose veins
5. gallbladder disease
6. endometriosis

---

true for women experiencing both natural and surgical meno-pause. If you are using HRT for osteoporosis prevention, you should start within the first few years after your last period.

Pre-HRT Evaluation

If you are considering taking hormone replacement therapy, you need to see a doctor for an evaluation and examination. The evaluation starts with a medical history. Certain circumstances under which you should not take HRT (contraindications) can be identified simply by answering a few questions.

The physical evaluation is similar to the examination done for a routine check up (see page 167). Blood tests are not routinely required before starting HRT. Sometimes an endometrial biopsy is done, particularly if you are in a high risk group for endometrial cancer (page 136) The test is invasive, painful and costly. Therefore only women suspected of having endometrial hyperplasia (overgrowth of the uterine lining) or of being at risk for endometrial cancer need a biopsy before beginning HRT. The frequency with which the biopsy is repeated should also be based on risk factors and symptoms. Unfortunately, doctors' fear of malpractice suits has increased their use of tests such as endometrial biopsy.

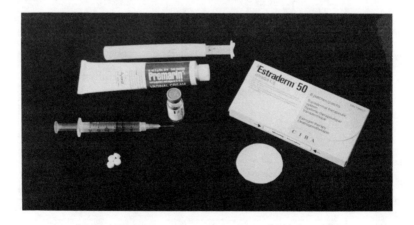

How To Take It

Hormone replacement therapy can be taken in many different ways. More research is needed to determine the best types of hormones, the best way to take them, the right amount, etc. In the meantime, there are many different dosages, forms and schedules. Most doctors familiarize themselves with one or two ways of prescribing hormones and stick with those. Many doctors keep up with the latest literature; others do not. Some like to experiment with new treatments; others need to see the results of many studies before they change the way they do things. Many decisions, such as the amount of progesterone in HRT, are based more on tradition than on scientific proof.

WAYS TO TAKE HRT

The most common way to take HRT is in pill form, but other ways of taking the treatment do exist. One advantage to other routes is that they avoid the digestive tract with its acids and enzymes which break down the hormones, as well as the liver which chemically changes them. Therefore you can get effective blood levels of the drug with a lower dose of medication. Also, avoiding the liver decreases the risk of liver and gallbladder complications.

Regardless of how you take them, the hormones are always absorbed into your blood stream and therefore have both the same effects and the same side effects as oral hormones.

The alternate routes are for the most part newer than oral HRT, and some are not yet available everywhere in North America.

Progesterone is still necessary even if the estrogen is taken in a form other than pills.

ESTROGEN CREAM is inserted into the vagina with an applicator marked for dosage. It is absorbed into the blood stream through the vaginal mucous membranes, but the precise dosage which ends up in the blood stream is hard to control. Estrogen cream has a local lubricating effect on the vagina as well.

INJECTIONS of estrogen, depo-provera and testosterone are available. The estrogen shot is effective for 4 to 6 weeks, depo-

(Continued)

141

The most common way to take HRT is in pill form (see insert for other ways to take it). You take estrogen once a day, for the first 25 days of the month. Progesterone is added for the last 10 days of estrogen treatment, i.e. from days 16 to 25. The last 5 or 6 days of the month, days 26 to 30 or 31, you take no pills at all. On the first of the month you start the process again, with estrogen only.

The dose of estrogen used depends on various factors such as your reason for taking the therapy, your body size, etc. The rule of thumb is to start with the lowest possible dose and then adjust up as necessary, rather than start high and adjust down.

Premarin, the most commonly prescribed estrogen, is available in .3 mg (green), .625 mg (maroon), .9 mg (white), 1.25 mg

---

(Continued)

provera works for three months, and testosterone is usually taken monthly. A combined estrogen/testosterone injection can be given every 4 weeks. The major disadvantage to hormones by injection is that if you develop side effects after having the injection, the effects cannot be reversed. Also, they require regular medical visits which can be costly as well as inconvenient.

HORMONE IMPLANTS are available in the U.S. but not in Canada. Implanting them involves minor surgery. The doctor cuts into the skin using a local anesthetic and inserts the pellet. The effects last for a few months. Both estrogen and testosterone are available in pellet form.

The ESTROGEN WAFER melted under the tongue is relatively new and not well known. The mouth and the mucous membranes under the tongue easily absorb estrogen into the blood stream. The wafer is not swallowed so the hormones do not pass by the liver and digestive system.

The TRANSDERMAL PATCH is a form of estrogen recently approved for use in North America. Patches are applied to the body twice weekly and the hormone is absorbed through the skin. The spot where the patch is applied should be rotated, and it should not be applied to the breasts. Redness can occur at the site of the patch.

142

(yellow) and 2.5 mg (purple). The most common starting dose is .625 mg because it is believed to be the minimum amount needed to prevent bone loss. If you are not taking the therapy to prevent osteoporosis, you can start with a lower dose. Provera (medroxyprogesterone acetate), the most common progesterone in use, is available in pills of 5 mg. The chart on page 144 lists other common hormones and their dosages.

You will probably have bleeding at some point during the 5 days you are off all pills. This is the withdrawal bleeding mentioned earlier. Some doctors are experimenting with giving progesterone only every third month so that you would only bleed every three months. It is not known how much and how often the endometrial lining has to be shed to limit the risks of endometrial cancer. If you have had a hysterectomy you will have no bleeding at the end of the cycle.

If you have had a hysterectomy you cannot get endometrial cancer. Therefore you can take estrogen continuously without having to stop for a week each month. Because progesterone is prescribed to decrease the risk of endometrial cancer it is not necessary to take it if your uterus has been removed, although some doctors do prescribe it.

Testosterone is a hormone produced by both men and women which increases sexual desire. In women, most testosterone is produced in the ovaries, even after menopause. Therefore if you have a surgical menopause you have less testosterone than women who still have their ovaries. If you have a decreased interest in sex after your surgery, you may be advised to take testosterone and estrogen together, either in pill or injection form. The most common side effect of this treatment is the growth of excess body hair. Little is known about the long-term effects of treatment with testosterone.

Follow-Up

The timing of the first follow-up visit to the doctor depends on whether you have any known risk factors for developing

COMMON BRANDS OF HORMONES USED IN HRT

TRADE NAMES	GENERIC NAMES	DAILY DOSE
Estrogen (oral)		
premarin	conjugated estrogen	3-1.25.mg
ogen	estropipate	.625-5 mg
estinyl	ethanyl estradiol	.2-.5 mg
tace	chlorotrianisene	12-25 mg
estrace	estradiol	1-2 mg
climestrone	esterified estrogen	1.25-3.75 mg
Estrogen (creams)		
premarin cream	conjugated estrogen	2-4 g
D.V. cream	dienestrol	1-2 applicators
Estrogen with Tranquilizers		
menrium	esterified estrogen & chlordiazepoxide	2-5 g estrogen 5-10 mg chlor.
Estrogen with Testosterone		
premarin with methyltestosterone	conjugated estrogen & methyltestosterone	.625-1.25 mg est. & 5-10 mg
climacterone	testosterone & estra-diol in oil	injection
estrand	estradiol valerate & testosterone enanthate	injection
Progestin		
provera	medroxyprogesterone acetate	5-10 mg
norlutate	norethindrone acetate	5 mg
micronor	norethindrone	.35-.7 mg

complications and on whether you experience any side effects. Usually it is scheduled for 3 to 6 months after starting treatment.

The follow-up visit is a time to discuss how things are going. How are you feeling on the hormones? Have you noticed any changes which might be indicative of a problem? Have the symptoms for which you started taking the hormones disappeared? If the treatment is not working, the dose can be adjusted. The same is true if it is causing inconvenient side effects. At that first visit and all future visits the doctor will check your blood pressure.

Subsequent follow-up visits are scheduled at 6 to 12 month intervals, depending on your doctor's usual practice and whether you are known to be at risk for complications, especially endometrial cancer. They follow the same format as the first visit and include a routine gynecological exam and a breast exam.

A D&C or aspiration will be proposed if you are having mid-cycle bleeding (bleeding while on the hormones), but is not necessary if you are having withdrawal bleeding (during the 5 days off the hormones). These procedures are described on page 101.

There is debate about how often, if at all, women who do not have mid-cycle bleeding should have endometrial biopsies. A commonly recommended protocol is to do them every 3 to 5 years, but these numbers are somewhat arbitrary. It is important to discuss each situation as it arises to see if an endometrial biopsy is actually necessary.

Regardless of the proposed follow-up schedule, you should consult a doctor at any point should you develop complications such as vaginal bleeding, abdominal pain, headaches, leg pain, etc.

Stopping HRT

The decision to stop taking HRT is made for different reasons and at different points in the treatment. Health problems or serious side effects may force you to stop. You may only have planned to use it for a short time, or you may get fed up with taking pills day after day or of monthly period-like bleeding.

When you stop the medication your hot flashes may return temporarily. Try to wean yourself from the hormones by taking only one half of the pill for at least two weeks before stopping. Give yourself a month at least before deciding whether or not the flashes are tolerable without hormones. Don't forget some of the non-drug strategies for dealing with flashes (page 60).

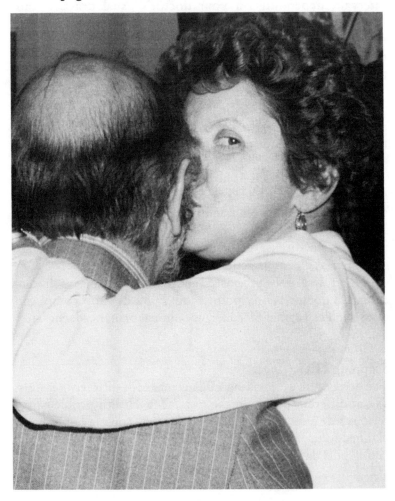

If you were taking HRT to help with discomfort from vaginal changes, you need to know that they will return eventually since they, unlike hot flashes, are long-term changes. The improvements brought about by the hormones will last for a while, but eventually you may have to look at other remedies if you stop HRT.

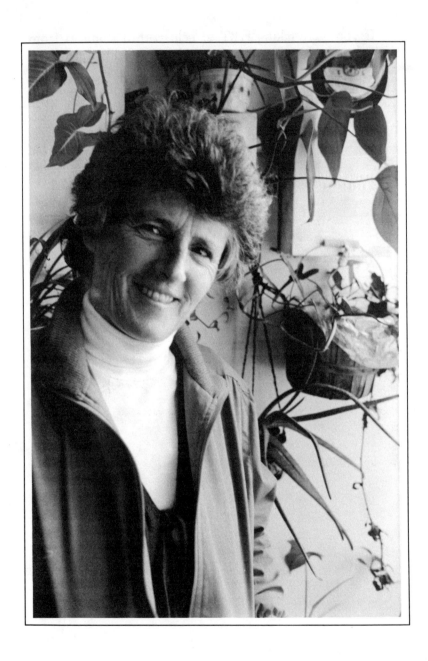

PART FOUR

LIVING HEALTHY LIVES

SEXUALITY IN THE MIDDLE YEARS AND BEYOND

One of the many myths about menopause is that it marks the end of sexual responsiveness — that it "neuters" women. In fact, we can be and often are sexually active well into old age. Each of us relates sexually to menopause in an individual and personal way. Our sexual ideas, preferences, desires and expectations affect our sex lives after menopause as they did before. They develop in response to many factors including our socio-cultural milieu, biology and personal experience of sexuality.

"I think it's [sexual desire] increasing. It's been at a low ebb for a while because I've been down. When you're feeling depressed and wiped out you don't feel like sex. I feel now the pleasure has increased. The orgasms seem stronger again. It was strong in adolescence and then there was a real dip when I was having my babies. In my early 30s

there was an increase again, then another dip. And now it's increased again. It surprised me."

Social Issues

The way we feel about ourselves as vital sexual beings has an impact on our libido, and our self-image is influenced by societal attitudes. By and large these attitudes have been ageist (prejudice based on age), sexist (prejudice based on gender) and puritanical (prejudice against sex itself).

We are led to believe that our aging bodies are undesirable. The 1986 model of the year was a 14-year-old from Toronto. *Vogue* presented her in a large photo layout entitled "the modern woman, fit and active." This "modern" woman, with a body unmarked by age, childbirth and the stresses of modern life, was presented as a realistic representation of mature womanhood. We are, on the other hand, beginning to see some signs of change. A television show like "The Golden Girls," with the incomparable Blanche Devereaux, would have been unthinkable 15 years ago.

Women who are 50 today came of age at a time when we were expected to repress our sexuality. Yet despite the prevailing norms, many of us have been able to claim our sexuality. We have had satisfying sex lives throughout our young adult years and expect to remain sexual well into old age.

Those involved in long-term relationships at mid-life may be redefining our roles within the couple or revitalizing an ailing marriage. If the relationship has generally worked, chances are it will continue to work. However, couples can fall into unsatisfying habits with each other which are hard to break. At times our sexual needs are not in sync with our partner's, causing tension in the relationship. Middle age is a good time to examine our relationships, to look at who we have become, to remember why we came together in the first place. Couples with sexual problems might choose to see a marriage counsellor or sex therapist to help sort out some of the tension and find some solutions.

One concern often mentioned by women whom we interviewed is the lack of available partners. In the menopausal years many of us are single due to divorce or separation. Others outlive our mates, without outliving our sexual desires and needs. Women live an average of 8 years longer than men. Divorced and widowed men tend to marry younger women. So the choice of male partners is more limited as we approach our 50s and 60s and beyond. (Lesbian women definitely come out ahead here, with a better chance of holding on to their mates into old age!)

Celibacy is often a reality after divorce, separation or the death of a partner. Some of us choose to remain celibate for the rest of our days and are satisfied with the affection and support of friends and family. Others would prefer to find a new partner with whom we can enjoy a sexual liaison. We have a number of options open to us.

Younger men are sometimes interested in older, mature women. A middle-aged woman can teach a young man about sex. We may not notice when a younger man is attracted to us because we think it could only happen to someone else — a woman with lots of money, power or prestige. That is a myth; April-December romances can be a nice surprise later in life.

Regardless of whether or not we have an available partner, one way that we can continue to remain sexual is through masturbation. Some of us are more comfortable than others taking this route, some more experienced at it than others. One nice thing about masturbation is that no one knows as well as we do ourselves, what kind of touching feels good and what gives us pleasure.

"It's hard to say whether menopause is causing any changes. If your sexual relationships are not constant you

don't know if it's your desire or whether this is really great or if you forgot how to do it and have to practice a few times. I think in general I have never felt better."

Biology

Our whole bodies are sexual. Sight, smell and touch are part of our sensory system, and love, lust and desire are complex reactions to the stimulation of our senses. Sexual desire grows and diminishes in response to all sorts of stimuli. A hand brushing a cheek, a twinkle in an eye or a smell that brings back memories can arouse all of us at one time or another.

Desire is also very much influenced by our minds and moods. Grief, anger, fear, guilt and sadness affect our sexual desire.

During the reproductive years, many of us feel more sexual at certain stages of our menstrual cycle, suggesting that hormones play a role too. Testosterone is considered to be closely linked with sexual desire. Estrogen seems to have the opposite effect, as many women who have taken high-dose birth control pills can attest. Therefore, the lower estrogen levels of the post-menopausal years combined with relatively higher testosterone levels may act to maintain or even increase our interest in sex as we get older.

The study of human sexuality is relatively new. It maps and examines physical responsiveness which is linked to emotions and is intimately personal. Scientists can measure our arousal by monitoring our heart beat and the blood flow to our genitals, but no one else can know our desire.

Researchers have divided human sexual response into four stages: excitement, plateau, climax and resolution. In reality these stages flow into each other, but this division is useful in trying to understand sexuality. As you go through menopause and the years following, you may experience changes in your sexual response related to the physical changes of menopause.

There are, for example, differences in the four stages of sexual arousal.

❖

"The only difference is lubrication."

❖

Excitement. During the excitement stage the heart and breathing rate increase. The skin may flush. The breasts enlarge and the nipples become erect. The clitoris also becomes erect and the inner labia swell and deepen in colour. The lining of the vagina releases a lubricating fluid. The deeper part of the vaginal walls separates and the uterus moves up in the pelvis, increasing the vaginal diameter.

After menopause you may get turned on more or less easily. Lubrication may take longer and there may be less of it depending on your estrogen levels. Your desire may be linked to your testosterone levels.

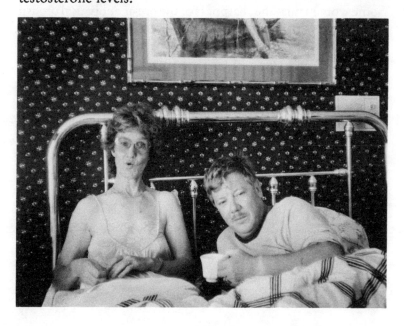

Plateau. If sexual stimulation continues, the body continues to respond. During the plateau stage, the heart rate and breathing become even faster. Muscle contraction and congestion in the pelvic area increase. The clitoris becomes exquisitely sensitive and retracts under the hood above it. Swelling of the vaginal opening decreases the diameter of the opening itself.

Some of these sensations may be less pronounced after menopause. Your heartbeat, breathing and blood pressure will still increase and you will experience the same muscular tension and excitement, but your nipples may not enlarge as much as during the reproductive years. Internally, vaginal engorgement and expansion may decrease. You may not even be aware of these subtle differences.

Orgasm. The sudden release of congestion and muscle tension is called orgasm or climax. The muscles at the vaginal opening contract and relax rhythmically. After menopause the pulsing pelvic and vaginal contractions can be slower and less intense. Some women miss the sharpness of the pre-menopausal orgasm and need time to readjust to these new sensations. Some women experience painful uterine contractions at orgasm after menopause.

Resolution. At resolution, the blood flow is released and the erect tissues lose their rigidity. If there is no further stimulation, the body returns to its normal state. There may be a thin film of sweat covering the body.

Some women are more orgasmic in their post-menopause; resolution takes longer and with little effort they can experience several orgasms in a row.

Any pain or discomfort during sex can decrease or extinguish your desire. So might hot flashes, flooding or depression. Fortunately, many sexual problems which may arise after menopause can be resolved. The first step is to understand the source of the problem.

154

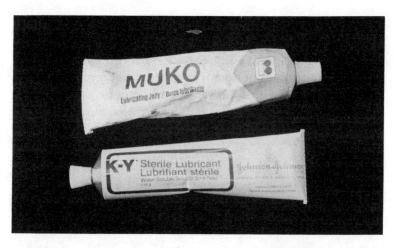

Having intercourse before you are well lubricated may cause vaginal pain or light bleeding. Part 2 discusses the vaginal changes after menopause and solutions to problems that can result.

If your vagina has shortened in length, your partner's thrusting penis may knock against your cervix. For some women this enhances their excitement. Others find it uncomfortable. If it is a problem for you, you might try positions in which you are on top during intercourse, giving you more control over how deeply your partner thrusts. This may also help if a vaginal scar due to hysterectomy causes pain during intercourse (see page 114).

Some drugs change sexual desire or response. For example, tranquilizers, anti-hypertensives (drugs which lower blood pressure) and anti-histamines (drugs which control allergic reactions) actually lower responsiveness. People are not always told about this type of side effect. You should ask your doctor when you are being prescribed any new drug whether it will affect your sexuality.

Some health problems make sexual activity difficult or uncomfortable. If arthritis makes movement too painful, sitting up on pillows may be more comfortable. Severe spinal osteoporosis may make some positions impossible. You might try lying on your side, with your partner behind your back. If you have recently had a heart attack, you will receive specific information from your doctor or nurse about resuming sexual activity. Anyone with a new illness may require time to adjust to their new reality before resuming sexual activity.

"I don't know what is the connection with the hysterectomy, but I know I easily get bladder infections when I get involved sexually."

Personal Experience

"I have no more interest in sex. Not with my husband or with another man. It's been two years."

Sexual appetites vary from individual to individual. The sexual side of a person's life is private and personal. Some of us are sexually timid while others are bold. We may have had a great deal of sexual experience with many different partners or remained with one steady partner for many years. Some of us initiate sex play, while others want their partner to make the first move. Some couples have passionate sex lives while others do not. Some of us will be sexually active into our 90s, as unlikely as that may seem to our children. Feeling turned on, desirous and desirable does not necessarily change just because we are older.

The women we interviewed in preparing this book varied greatly one from another regarding their sexuality. Some had an increased interest in sex after menopause. Others, for whom sex had never been fulfilling, found that at menopause, they preferred to close that chapter in their lives. Many talked about having held themselves back sexually because of the constant threat of an unwanted pregnancy or because of the demands of a young family. Now when the demands and risks are different, they are experiencing an awakening of libido which is surprising and exciting. Women who had always related their sexuality to reproduction talked about a loss of sexual desire after menopause. Others were still interested but had difficulty finding partners or were no longer interested in trying new relationships, although they still felt sexual desires and urges. We will know more about menopause and sexuality when women and men feel more comfortable talking about it. This exchange will probably confirm the same healthy variety of experiences for mid-life women as for younger women.

"I don't know whether it is due to the hysterectomy or due to the therapy, but I started to just move ahead and have one affair, two affairs and then a very ongoing affair for the past twelve years. Now whether it has something to do with the freedom that came with the fact that it would no longer be dangerous — to be illegitimately pregnant. I know that I started to get involved after the surgery."

Birth Control Around Menopause
As menopause approaches and ovulation becomes more irregular, we become less fertile — that is, less likely to become pregnant. Irregular periods make it difficult to predict when we are fertile, and we cannot use a missed period as an indicator of pregnancy the way we did before. Pregnancy scares cause great anxiety when we know we are taking contraceptive risks. Thus, if we are sexually active, we need a birth control method that feels comfortable and inspires confidence. We should use some

method of birth control for 12 to 24 months after our last period. This advice is often difficult to follow. Although by mid-life most of us are pretty clear about not wanting another child, our knowledge that we are less fertile and less likely to get pregnant makes it tempting to be less vigilant.

Some women who start missing periods do occasional

BIRTH CONTROL ISSUES FOR MID-LIFE WOMEN

Birth Control Pill
Age & cigarette smoking act together to increase the risk of side effects. Not usually prescribed after age 35 for smokers, 40 for non-smokers.

IUD
Thought to present less risk of pelvic infection and pain in older women who have had a baby. Women with flooding may find the heavier periods associated with IUD to be a problem.

Barrier Methods
(condoms, spermicides, diaphragm, cervical cap and sponge)
If pelvic relaxation exists, a good fit for a diaphragm is not always possible.

Calendar (rhythm)
Not reliable due to irregular cycle.

Sympto-thermic
(combined basal body temperature and examination of cervical secretions)
May be more difficult to use due to erratic cycles, to long stretches between ovulations and to the effect of hormonal changes on cervical mucus.

Sterilization
No special problems vis-a-vis tubal ligation. Hysterectomy should not be used as a means of sterilization.

Morning-After Pill
No special problems.

pregnancy tests. The hormone changes of menopause can cause false positive tests (that is, the test is positive but the woman is not pregnant). Any positive test should be confirmed by a physical examination.

If you are taking hormone replacement therapy you still need to use birth control. The doses of estrogen and progesterone in HRT are not high enough to prevent ovulation.

Some birth control issues for pre-menopausal women are unique. However, in general, the questions faced by women who must make contraceptive choices are the same regardless of age. They are: the effectiveness of the method in preventing pregnancy; the possible side effects; the impact on sexuality; and the cost. The one factor which is no longer an issue for us as mid-life women is the reversibility of the method, that is, whether it might prevent us from getting pregnant in the future.

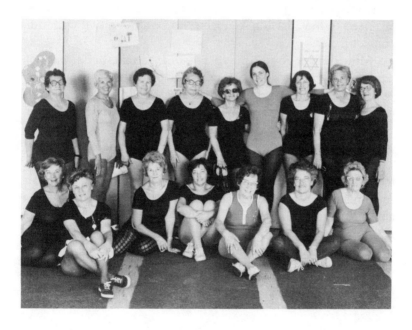

TAKING CARE OF OURSELVES

*"I feel that we tamper so much with our natural biology
that we lose touch really. And every now and again we are
forced to look at our bodies and their function. Menopause
is sort of a time to take stock."*

Most of what we cope with during the mid-life years —
including menopause — are not medical problems but life
issues. To take care of ourselves during this period, some
medical knowledge certainly helps. But the experience we have
accumulated during 50 years of life is equally important. So are
the experiences that other women have had and are willing to
share with us. Taking care of ourselves requires certain lifestyle
decisions: to eat well or not, to exercise or be sedentary, to stop
smoking or give up the battle. We live with many competing
pressures, doing the best we can under our own circumstances.
We need to have faith in ourselves to be able to live with our
compromises.

Mid-life is a good time to organize to take better care of
ourselves. It coincides with the shift of focus from meeting
others' needs to meeting our own. We can do many things to
help keep our minds and bodies in smooth running order
before problems arise. We need not wait until we are run down
or sick to invest energy in ourselves and our bodies.

We can start by simply devoting a bit more time to being in
touch with ourselves, what we need, how we are feeling. We can
re-think the habits that affect our health and make decisions
about changing our lifestyle. We can expand and strengthen our
relationships with family and friends, and link up with groups
in our communities that share our interests and needs. Support
systems such as these give us a sense of belonging, essential to
our health. They also provide a means of meeting new people,

something that can become more difficult as we get older. These kinds of actions will not necessarily protect us from illness. Many other factors contribute to illness — our genetic make-up, our economic conditions, the environmental and

---

LIFESTYLE ISSUES

Smoking:
Most people know that cigarette smoking is related to lung and heart disease. Fewer are aware that women who smoke (or whose partner smokes) may go through menopause earlier than those who don't.

Although fewer people smoke today, young women smoke in greater numbers than before.

Smoking is an addiction. Quitting requires will power, courage and support. Take advantage of places where smoking is forbidden. Find out what services are offered in your community for people who want to quit. Don't be discouraged if you've tried before without success. Statistics show that your chances of succeeding improve with each attempt. You'll know when you find an approach that's right for you - because it works!

Alcohol:
Light drinking relaxes us and may be associated with a decrease in heart disease. However heavy drinking causes serious health problems as well as social and economic difficulties. Moderate drinking is related to accidents and has a possible link with breast cancer.

Each of us should take stock of our drinking habits. How much money do we spend on drinking? Are most of our friends drinking buddies? How often do we change our plans because of a hangover? Should we be cutting back?

Fewer services exist for women alcoholics, who are often treated with tranquilizers before the real problem is discovered. If you have a problem with alcohol, go to a person or group experienced in helping people with alcohol problems.

Physical Activity:
For most of us, our regular daily activities are not a good enough workout to keep our bodies in shape. Many of us have trouble

(Continued)

---

occupational hazards that we face. To focus only on our bad habits is to take a narrow approach which fails to address these other issues. But to blame society and absolve ourselves is not more useful. Lifestyle changes and greater attention to our-

---

(Continued)

making that extra effort to exercise regularly.

The benefits of exercise are well known: our bodies are more flexible. We sleep better and have a more positive self image.

It is never too late to begin exercising. Older people can improve their strength, endurance and cardiovascular condition just as much as younger people. Some Y's and health clubs provide work-out programs geared to the needs of middle-aged people, as well as programs for people who are just beginning to exercise after years of inactivity.

Many women never participated in sports and feel awkward beginning in mid-life. Find an activity you enjoy and start gradually. You may be surprised how well you do!

Eating:

Everyone needs to eat but we each relate to food differently. Can we afford fresh food? Do we have time to enjoy preparing a meal? Do we skip meals and guiltily nibble snacks instead? Is food a reward? Are we too lonely to eat?

Learning what to eat is easy. Government guidelines suggest portions from each of the four food groups which contain the basic nutrients we need. Organizing our lives to eat well is more difficult. It takes a certain commitment to resist the fast food temptation. Many people are finding the return to good eating to be the solution to some health problems.

Feeding the Soul:

Not only our stomachs need to be fed! Human beings have lots of less tangible needs - security, affection, harmony, a sense of being useful and creative, etc. We try to make some sense of the universe and our place in it. We need to stay in touch with ourselves and each other.

We have fewer rituals to help us integrate life's events and stages. Many feel awkward with meditation, prayer or even play. It is important for each of us to find some interest or activity that renews the spirit and restores the soul.

---

selves and our health may, in some cases, prevent illness. More important, they contribute to our health by helping us to function at a higher capacity. We may feel more energetic and better about our lives.

This way of caring for ourselves is what the women's health movement calls self help. It has been part of the movement since the early 1970s when women first started learning to use a speculum to help them get to know their bodies, and experimenting with home remedies for common gynecological problems.

Self help as we use it in this book is based on the same principle — that we know ourselves best and that in many situations we have the capacity to take care of and heal ourselves. This is a holistic concept which extends beyond gynecological issues. It can take many forms ranging from herbal remedies for menstrual pain to relaxation exercises, from joining a support group with other mid-life women to taking up square dancing.

WELL WOMAN CARE

"I think women should know everything about their own bodies. They should be taught from early childhood how it functions. If the interest is not developed early the tendency is not to bother with it. I pride myself on being intelligent but I was not knowledgeable and I did not ask the right questions. We have to take much more responsibility for ourselves."

Even as we care for ourselves, we can also take advantage of the health care system and the resources it offers. Consulting a health care professional when we are well is referred to as well woman care. It can help us prevent illness and improve our health and the quality of our lives.

Well woman care should consist of a check-up, screening tests and health education. If the visit is superficial and limited only to a gynecological exam, we aren't really getting our money's worth. It is education that gives us the tools we need to assert control over our health. The knowledge and insight we gain from well woman care may ultimately have more of an impact on our health than a physical examination or a blood test.

Frequency

Unless a problem or complication requires more frequent visits, you should see a health practitioner once a year. If you are taking regular medication or are at risk of developing certain problems, you might need to go more often.

Settings

The type and quality of care you receive is influenced by both the practitioner and the setting you choose. Each has its advantages and disadvantages. Factors to consider include the general atmosphere, continuity of care, cost and whether you prefer a global approach to health or specialization.

A family doctor who knows your physical and social history might consider your more general health needs rather than focus on just one part of you. Of all the medical providers, family practitioners are the ones whose training most focuses on prevention and on aspects of health as well as illness. However not all family doctors are up to date on some of the more specialized aspects of well woman care such as birth control or hormone replacement therapy. Should you develop serious problems, you will be referred to a specialist.

Often we choose an obstetrician/gynecologist when we are pregnant and then stay with that doctor for routine care. Because we are encouraged to have regular Pap smears and require medical visits for birth control, we continue to see the

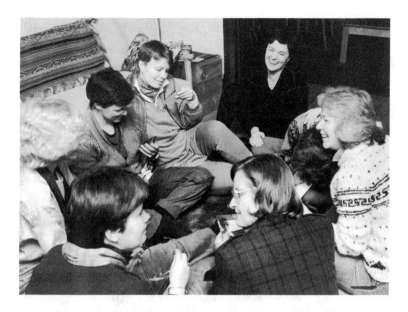

gynecologist regularly, and consider that visit as our annual check-up. Sometimes that is the only doctor we see.

Gynecologists are specialists whose training prepares them to deal with specialized problems. They may be more up to date on the latest research and practice in some areas, but preventive care to healthy women is less interesting to them. The care they provide may not be satisfactory if they are not interested in answering questions and giving explanations. Since gynecology focuses primarily on the reproductive system, we will be referred to another doctor if we have other kinds of problems. We may end up feeling that no one person is really looking after us.

Community clinics and women's health centres often hold a specific philosophy of care which emphasizes education and encourages women to be involved in decision-making about their own health. Nurses and lay health workers play an important role in these settings. However you might not see the same doctor at each visit.

Hospital clinics tend to be impersonal, with an almost assembly-line style. At a teaching hospital you will likely be seen by a medical student. But hospitals sometimes offer specialized clinics and equipment that may not be available elsewhere.

The rest of this chapter describes a routine well woman care visit. Its purpose is to explain some of the usual procedures and to set a standard by which you can judge the quality of the service you are receiving.

The Consultation

Personal History. You will be asked to talk about your health: major illnesses, hospitalizations, operations, medication you take regularly, and any new symptoms. You will be asked a series of questions about each body system (for example, digestion), with a special emphasis on identifying specific problems for which you are at risk due to your age, lifestyle or family history. If you are unclear about the diagnosis or treatment of any illness, you can ask that a summary of your previous charts be sent to your doctor. You should mention any regular habits, such as cigarettes and alcohol, or special diet, and give a brief account of your responsibilities — job, family, school, recreation — and your feelings about them.

Health problems of other members of your family which could be relevant to your own health should be noted, for example high blood pressure, diabetes, cancer, etc.

You describe your reproductive history. At what age did you begin having menstrual periods? Are you still having them? If so, have they changed over the past few years? In what way? How often do you get periods? How long does the bleeding last and how heavy is it? Do you have any bleeding between periods or after intercourse? If you are no longer having periods, when did they stop? Do you have hot flashes or other symptoms of menopause? If you are nearing menopause and have been keeping a menstrual chart, you can discuss it with the doctor. You will also be asked about your pregnancies and their outcomes — miscarriage, induced abortion, or delivery. You may discuss your sexual experience, in particular your present experience(s). Do you have one partner or several? Are you satisfied with your sex life? If not, what do you see as the problem? Are you finding that vaginal changes associated with menopause are affecting your sex life? If you still require contraception (have had a period in the past 1–2 years), you can discuss the method you are presently using, problems you have had with it and reasons you might want to change methods.

Physical Examination. Some of us are nervous about physical examinations. We must expose our bodies to the sight and touch of a stranger, often male. As we get older we may begin to feel odd seeing a doctor, particularly a male doctor, who is 20 or more years younger than we are.

The gynecological examination ("pelvic") may especially cause anxiety. After 30 years of pelvic exams, some of us are as comfortable with them as we are climbing on a bicycle. Others are still nervous. The more you relax, the more useful and the less uncomfortable this examination is. Usually the examination is not painful. Pain is caused by tension, rough handling or disease. It is the examiner's responsibility to help you relax.

If you are going to have a pelvic exam, you should not use douches, creams or powders for at least 24 hours beforehand as they can hide signs of infection. The examination will be more comfortable if you empty your bladder beforehand.

You will weigh yourself. Your height is measured and blood pressure taken. A brief examination should be made of all your body systems and any problem area is examined more thoroughly. A breast examination is done. If you do not know how to examine your own breasts, you should be taught how.

For a pelvic examination, your outer genitals are examined first. The doctor looks for signs of irritation, suspicious growths and pelvic relaxation.

As part of the pelvic exam the muscles that support your pelvic floor and hold your uterus, bladder and rectum in place will be checked for signs of prolapse, i.e. the bulging of these organs through weakened pelvic floor muscles.

To look inside your vagina and at your cervix, the examiner uses a metal or plastic speculum. A metal speculum should be warmed first and both kinds should be lubricated with water or jelly. After menopause your vaginal walls may be thin and less well lubricated, so special care should be taken to insert the speculum gently and not to cause pain during the exam. The speculum is inserted into the vagina with its blades closed, and the blades are then gently opened. The speculum is moved until your cervix can be clearly seen. The cervix of a woman at menopause looks paler than during the reproductive years. A Pap test or cytology for cervical cancer is done if needed.

To examine your internal organs (uterus, ovaries and Fallopian tubes), the examiner puts two fingers of a gloved hand into your vagina and puts the other hand on your lower abdomen. Your uterus can be felt between the two hands, but in post-menopausal women — and many pre-menopausal women — the ovaries are hard to find. If they appear enlarged, it could mean there is a problem and that further investigation should be done.

A rectal examination is done in women over 40 to detect early signs of rectal cancer. The examiner will insert one gloved finger into your rectum to feel for any lumps. You may feel some discomfort, as though you are going to have a bowel movement, especially when the finger is removed, but this will not happen.

Screening. Screening is a public health technique to distinguish between the majority of people who are healthy and the few who have problems as yet undetected. Further investigation and possible treatment are offered only to those who are found to have a problem. Well-known screening tests include the Pap

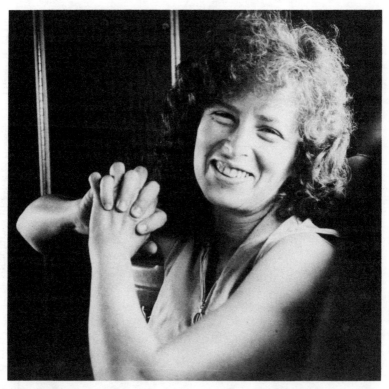

test for cervical cancer and the skin test for tuberculosis. Screening may consist of questions (for example, about working conditions), a physical examination (for example, for breast cancer) or laboratory tests (for example, the Pap test). When a person is ill, the same tests are used for diagnosis. This is no longer considered screening since the person already knows a problem exists.

Deciding who should be screened for a specific condition is not always easy. For screening to be appropriate the condition should be common and treatable and the test should be inexpensive and reliable. For example, screening for high blood pressure is useful because the test is simple and the illness is common and treatable.

169

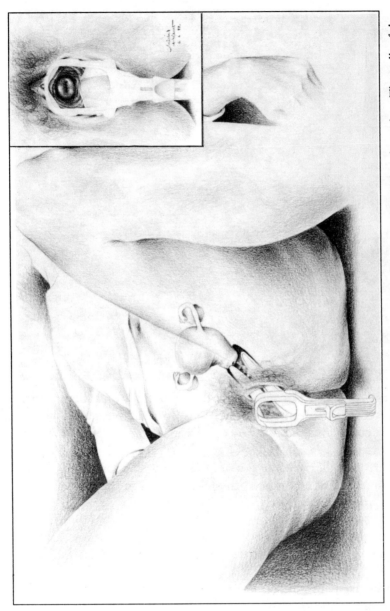

GYNECOLOGICAL EXAMINATION – A metal or plastic speculum is inserted in the vagina. The walls of the vagina and the cervix are examined. Inset: direct view of the cervix.

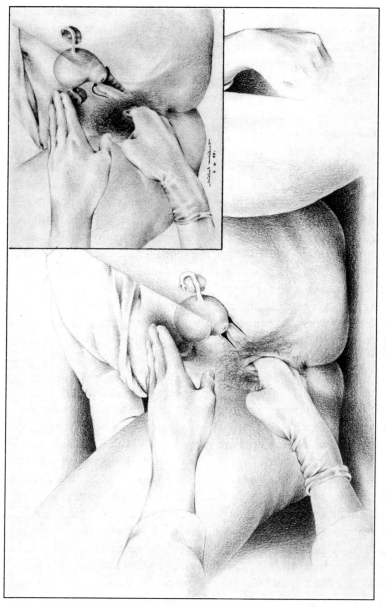

BIMANUAL EXAMINATION – With one hand on the abdomen and two fingers in the vagina, the examiner feels the uterus, noting its size, shape and position. Inset: examiner feels each ovary and tube.

Well woman care requires few tests. You should ask why a test is being ordered. You may have had a similar test recently or may feel it is not worth the money, either from your own pocket or the government's.

Tests that might be appropriate include urine tests to screen for kidney function or blood tests for anemia, diabetes, cholesterol or thyroid function. If you have more than one male sexual partner or your regular partner has other lovers, you should have tests done for sexually transmitted diseases such as gonorrhea, chlamydia (where tests are available), and possibly syphilis and AIDS.

Yearly Pap smears have been a cornerstone of routine gynecological care. But in 1979, a task force of the Canadian Medical Association recommended yearly Pap smears only for women at high risk for cervical cancer. These include women who had their first sexual relations at an early age, those with several partners and those with a history of sexually transmitted disease, in particular, venereal warts. Otherwise a Pap smear was recommended every 3 years up to the age of 35 and every 5 years after that so long as the most recent test was normal. In fact, the majority of women who consult doctors still have yearly Pap smears. Although these tests are not risky, they are costly. Probably too many Pap tests are done among urban and middle class women, and not enough among the rural and poor. This is an example of how many factors beyond just science influence what care a person gets.

Sometimes a screening test for intestinal bleeding is done on stool which remains on the examining glove after a rectal exam. This test, used as a preliminary screening for cancer of the intestines, often gives false positives (shows that there is blood in the stool when there really is not). This causes needless worry. A positive test should be repeated under more controlled conditions (for example, ensuring that there is no aspirin in your system), and only if it is still positive should other tests be done. If you have a family history of intestinal cancer you should have a more thorough evaluation every couple of years.

Sometimes electrocardiograms are prescribed for mid-life and older women to screen for heart disease. Since no evidence exists that these tests accurately predict who will have a heart attack, there is no need to have one if you are not having symptoms.

The use of mammography to screen for breast cancer is discussed on page 106. Screening for endometrial cancer is discussed on page 104.

Education. This is an important part of well woman care. It may be quite informal; when the blood pressure is taken, a simple explanation can be given of what blood pressure is. In some settings it may be more structured, with time set aside for you to ask questions and voice concerns. Education can be done by the same practitioner who examines you, or by someone else, usually a nurse or health educator.

Regardless of how your visit is organized, you should feel you have had all of your questions answered. You should understand why any tests or procedures are being done, as well as the implications of both positive and negative results. Be sure you understand what medications you are taking, why you are taking them, what the side effects might be and how long you should be on them. It is a good idea to review periodically with the doctor the medications you are taking to be sure you still need them.

If you are faced with a decision, such as whether to have surgery or whether to take hormone replacement therapy, you should have adequate information about the pros and cons and not feel rushed in your decision making. Feel free to ask for a second opinion about surgery or other major procedures.

Some of us find that we are more successful at getting our questions answered if we bring a list with us. You can also bring a friend or family member as an advocate or support person. When a lot of complex or frightening information is to be discussed, it is useful to have another person with you to hear it and to discuss and work it through with after the visit is over.

BREAST CARE

Menopause does not cause breast problems. In fact, it solves some of them. However, the increased risk of breast cancer as we get older forces us to take it into consideration. It is estimated that 1 out of 11 women will develop breast cancer in their lifetime. The fear of breast cancer creates great anxiety, as does the prospect of radical surgical treatments such as mastectomy (removal of a breast).

Common Non-Cancerous Breast Problems

Fibrocystic Breasts are the most common non-cancerous breast condition. It occurs primarily between the ages of 30 — 50 and resolves once menopause is over. It causes a thickening of breast tissue, breast pain and occasionally, fluid-filled cysts. The symptoms are linked to the menstrual cycle, getting worse just before each period and better once the period begins. Fibrocystic breasts are not a disease at all, but simply a variation of normal breast changes.

Types of fibrocystic breast conditions are classified according to microscopic differences. Only one of the less common types appears to be linked to an increased risk of cancer. Most women with fibrocystic breasts do not need to have a biopsy so they do not know which type they have.

Caffeine (coffee, tea, chocolate, cola) has been linked to fibrocystic breasts. While some studies have shown a clear link, others find no association between the two. Still, many women who eliminate or reduce their caffeine intake notice a decrease in both breast lumps and tenderness. There is no known relationship between caffeine and breast cancer.

Duct Ectasis (Comedomastitis) is a breast condition which occurs around the time of menopause, most commonly in women who have nursed babies. The symptoms are burning around the nipples, a sticky, multicolored nipple discharge from both nipples and sometimes a breast lump. There is no relationship between this condition and breast cancer, but they can be difficult to differentiate, and a biopsy may be necessary to make the diagnosis.

Intraductal Papilloma occurs most often in women between the ages of 35 and 45. The main symptom is a liquid, sometimes bloody discharge from one nipple. The usual treatment is to surgically remove the duct that is affected, removing about ½ centimeter of breast tissue.

Screening For Breast Cancer
The purpose of screening programmes is to detect breast cancer early in order to increase the possibility of curing the disease or at least of increasing the number of years that a woman will live after the disease has been diagnosed. The Canadian Cancer Society recommends that in addition to monthly breast self examination, women over the age of 50 should have a yearly mammogram (see page 106). The American Cancer Society is even more aggressive in its recommendations. A major study is in progress across Canada to determine the value of routine screening with mammography at different ages.

The belief that underlies intensive screening of women without symptoms is that those who develop cancer will live longer if it is caught early. However survival rates for breast cancer have not improved significantly over the past 50 years in spite of screening programs and more sophisticated treatment methods. It is possible that different types of breast cancer exist, some of which rarely metastasize (spread to other parts of the body) and others that have probably already spread by the time even the smallest cancer is found. Breast cancers that occur

BREAST SELF EXAMINATION

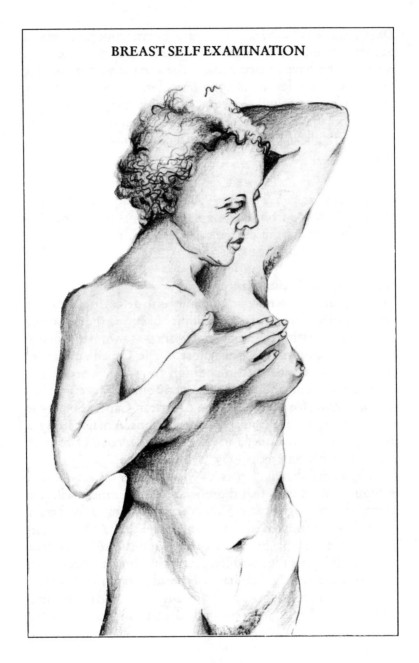

before menopause may be different from those that occur after.

The costs of regular screening with mammography are also a concern. These include unnecessary breast surgery because of false positive results, false reassurance in women who have negative results and therefore assume they are okay until the next mammography, increased anxiety about breast cancer in the entire population of women over 50, and finally, the very small but real risk associated with yearly radiation exposure to the breasts.

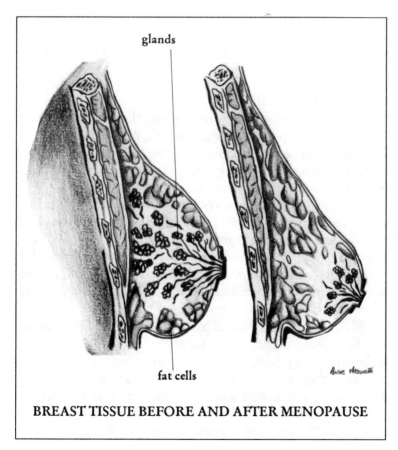

glands

fat cells

BREAST TISSUE BEFORE AND AFTER MENOPAUSE

In light of present knowledge, we are comfortable recommending that women between the ages of 50 and 60 have mammography yearly. So should women over 40 whose mother or sister had breast cancer. For other women between 40 and 50, and for women over 60, the evidence is less clear.

Mammography should be done in a centre which has modern equipment (that emits less radiation) and whose staff has the experience necessary to interpret the films. When possible, it is preferable to return to the same place so that this year's test can be compared to earlier ones.

Mammography is still an important and very useful test for diagnosis when symptoms of breast problems exist. A complete discussion of the treatment of breast cancer is beyond the scope of this book.

Breast Self Examination

In breast self examination, women check their own breasts on a monthly basis to look for breast lumps. Approximately 85% of all breast cancers are discovered by the woman herself or her lover, sometimes while doing an examination, other times while making love, getting dressed, etc.

Although the controversy around screening for breast cancer applies to self examination as well, it is probably a good habit to develop. No risks are involved with it. It allows you the opportunity to learn more about and feel more comfortable with your body. Also, although there is some doubt as to whether early detection actually increases cure rates, it may allow you more treatment options.

Many of us are frightened by breast self exam. Often we do not do it — either because we are scared or because we cannot be bothered. Try doing it in the shower or bath. If your hands are soapy they will glide over your breasts and make the exam easier. Some women find it helps to close their eyes and let their fingers "see" for them. About 80% of breast lumps are not cancerous. With regular self examination you will get to know the contours of your own breasts. The exam becomes easier and less stressful over time.

Both the Canadian and American Cancer Societies distribute pamphlets describing the technique of breast self examination. You can also ask your health care provider if you are not sure whether you are doing it correctly.

POSTSCRIPT

*"I feel I have 20 years to do things for me. In my mind I feel
that by my 70s I'll be more vulnerable, less ready to take
risks. So I have lots of energy to do things now."*

In the preparation of this book an important debate took place
around how much to include on the subject of aging. We found
that we had to resist falling into the trap of discussing menopause as if it were part of being old, rather than part of mid-life.
We started to write a chapter about the plight of elderly women
— about their high rate of poverty, their living conditions, the
effects of sexism and of the stereotypes about the elderly with
regard to work, mental capacities and sexuality.

As work progressed, we recognized that while the issues
raised by the chapter were serious and very real, they belonged
in another book — one about women and aging. With the life
expectancy for women approaching 80, the links between
menopause and old age are tenuous.

We do feel strongly that as mid-life women we need to
know what is ahead. We are at a point in our lives at which we
can make crucial plans and decisions which will affect us as we

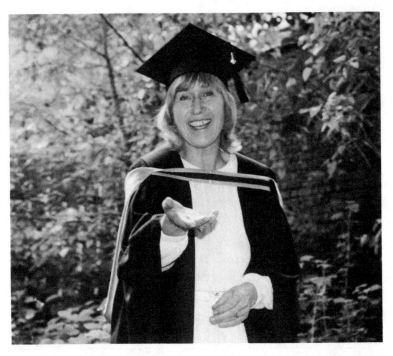

get older. To plan for old age while we are still middle-aged is no different from taking prenatal and parenting classes while we are still pregnant, or teaching adolescents who are not yet sexually active about birth control and the responsibilities engendered by sexuality. It just makes good sense.

Planning for old age does not make us age faster. It is a gesture of maturity to recognize that we will not always be as independent as we are now. We want to assure our living conditions later on without creating an overwhelming burden for those close to us.

The most important area in which planning may make a difference is the area of finances. What is your financial status? If you have a pension plan, do you understand it? If you are married, do you know enough about your husband's finances — debts, savings, life insurance, will, pension plan, etc? Does your health insurance seem adequate?

Too many women find themselves alone, with little or no income, or widowed, without knowing what financial arrangements their husbands have made. Some divorced and widowed women do not know how to manage their regular finances; many more do not have enough money to manage. Although money cannot buy good health and happiness, it certainly goes a long way towards helping us secure the resources we need to live our lives with dignity and with our basic needs met. To try to assure that we will have the resources we need, we should start planning now.

Another important way that we can act now to enhance our later years is by working together to bring about change. The hardships faced by older women are not the result of personal failings, but of social and economic injustices which reflect society's prejudices against women and the elderly. Pension plans, for example, are not designed with the work patterns of women in mind. Women often spend fewer years in the paid work force, moving in and out when children are young, and on the average they tend to have lower incomes than their male

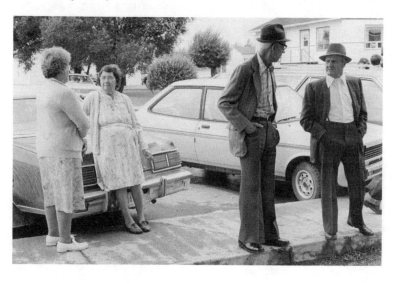

counterparts due to the wage gap. As a consequence, they have lower pensions and less ability to save, both factors that have a major impact on the conditions under which they live when they are older.

Many problems faced by these women will require a concerted effort to change, and that effort need not come only from the elderly themselves. The rest of us can also help to see that the interests of this group of women are heard and considered.

As the baby-boom generation hits mid-life and beyond, it will influence by its sheer numbers the experience of aging. In Canada by the year 2031, one person in 5 will be over 65 years old. This is a generation that expects to be heard and expects answers. Its members are experienced organizers, used to lobbying effectively, in their own interests and for more global social concerns. Baby boomers are used to challenging authority and to insisting on tolerance for a variety of lifestyles. Such an activist approach to life makes the future seem hopeful and exciting.

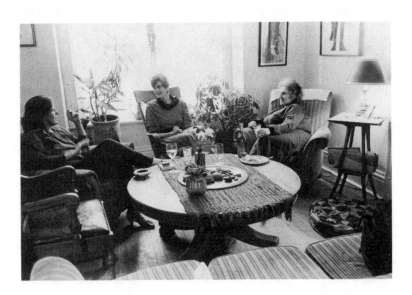

OTHER READING

BOOKS AND JOURNALS

Boston Women's Health Collective. *The New Our Bodies, Ourselves.* New York: Simon and Schuster,1984.

Cobb, Janine O'Leary. *Understanding Menopause.* Toronto: Key Porter Books, 1989.

Cutler, W. *Hysterectomy: Before and After.* New York: Harper and Row, 1988.

Cutler, W., Garcia, C.R. & Edwards, D. *Menopause: A Guide for Women and the Men Who Love Them.* New York: W.W. Norton,1983

Cutler, W., Garcia, C.R. *The Medical Management of Menopause and Premenopause.* Philadelphia: J.B. Lippincott, 1984.

Doress, P.B. & Siegal, D.L. *Ourselves Growing Older: Women Aging With Knowledge and Power.* New York: Simon & Schuster, 1987.

Greenwood, S. *Menopause Naturally.* San Fransisco: Volcano Press, 1984.

Hufnagel, V. *No More Hysterectomies.* New York: New American Library, 1988.

Kaufert, P.A. "Myth and the menopause." *Sociology of Health and Illness,* 4(2): 141-166, 1982.

MacPherson, K.I. "Menopause as disease: The social construction of a metaphor." *Advances in Nursing Science,* 3, 95-113, 1981.

McCrea, F.B. "The politics of menopause: The 'discovery' of a deficiency disease." *Social Problems*, 31(1), 111-123, 1983.

Morgan, S. *Coping with Hysterectomy* (rev. ed.). New York: New American Library, 1985.

National Women's Health Network. *Taking Hormones and Women's Health*. Washington D.C., 1989.

Porcino, J. *Growing Older, Getting Better*. Reading, Mass.: Addison-Wesley, 1983.

Reitz, Rosetta. *Menopause: A Positive Approach*. New York: Penguin Books, 1977.

Rubin, L. *Women of a Certain Age*. New York: Harper & Row, 1979.

Seaman, B., & Seaman, G. *Women and the Crisis in Sex Hormones*. New York: Bantam, 1977.

NEWSLETTERS AND PERIODICALS

A Friend Indeed. Box 515, Place du Parc Station, Montreal, Quebec H2V 2P1.

Broomstick: Options For Women Over 40. 3543 18th St. #3, San Francisco, California 94110.

Healthsharing. A Canadian Women's Health Quarterly. 14 Skey Lane, Toronto, Ontario M6J 3S4.

Hot Flash: Newsletter for Midlife and Older Women. Box 816, Stony Brook, N.Y. 11790-0609.

FILMS AND VIDEOS

Is It Hot In Here? L. Alper and H. Paul (1986). National Film Board of Canada. P.O. Box 6100, Montreal, Quebec H3C 3H5.

The Best Time Of My Life. P. Watson (1986). National Film Board of Canada. P.O. Box 6100, Montreal, Quebec H3C 3H5.

INDEX

The Montreal Health Press is a collective of women who write, publish and distribute handbooks about health and sexuality. They provide unbiased, non-judgmental information and encourage people to make their own personal decisions on these fundamental issues.

The Montreal Health Press was officially founded in 1972. But its early members had already made history in 1968, by publishing the Birth Control Handbook at a time when disseminating birth control information was still illegal in Canada.

The inexpensive format of the handbooks made mass distribution possible. Millions of copies have been provided to women through clinics, community centres, hospitals, women's groups, colleges and universities throughout North America.

Menopause: A Well Woman Book is the first of the handbooks to be published in book form. This reliable and reassuring health resource for women of the 1990s is now available to a new, wider audience.

The Montreal Health Press can be contacted at
P.O. Box 1000, Place du Parc, Montreal,
Quebec, Canada H2W 2N1

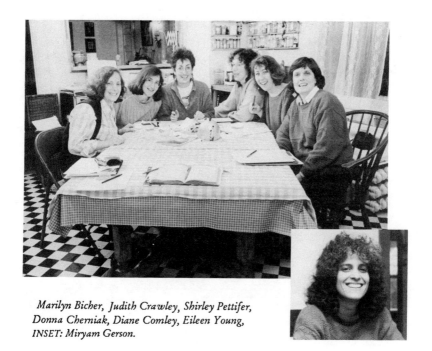

Marilyn Bicher, Judith Crawley, Shirley Pettifer, Donna Cherniak, Diane Comley, Eileen Young, INSET: Miryam Gerson.